Consciousness Reconnected

Missing links between self, neuroscience, psychology and the arts

Derek Steinberg

Formerly Consultant Psychiatrist and Clinical Teacher
The Maudsley and Bethlem Royal Hospitals, University of London

T0133939

Foreword by
Peter Tyrer

Illustrations by the author

Radcliffe Publishing
Oxford • Seattle

Radcliffe Publishing Ltd
18 Marcham Road
Abingdon
Oxon OX14 1AA
United Kingdom

www.radcliffe-oxford.com
Electronic catalogue and worldwide online ordering facility.

British Library Cataloguing in Publication data

A catalogue record for this book is available from the British Library.

ISBN-10 1 85775 778 5
ISBN-13 978 1 85775 778 1

Typeset by Advance Typesetting Ltd, Oxford
Printed and bound by TJ International Ltd, Padstow, Cornwall

For Gill, Kate, and Anna
and
for all the ancestors and descendants

Contents

Foreword   vii

Preface   ix

About the author   xi

Other books by Derek Steinberg   xii

Acknowledgements   xiii

1   A short walk around the subject   1

2   Consciousness disconnected   22
The title, some definitions, and ways of thinking about
consciousness

3   First stop Babel: advice before embarking   45
Tribal behaviour likely to be encountered during the excursions,
and how it throws light on the nature of consciousness

4   The genie in the genes: how chemicals could become
    conscious   53
How evolution and time led to a most extraordinary development

5   A fateful attachment   60
Family life: from necessities to niceties

6   Twists in the tale   90
Histories and mysteries: philosophies of mind and the uncertain
nature of reality

7   Archetype   102
Two serious heresies: the mystery of the archetype, and the
inheritance of experience

8   What the poets know   117
Art: the artist as visionary, magician, explorer and clown

9   Connecting up   139
    On making up one's mind

10 Clinical consciousness: a few notes   168
    Messages for psychiatry?

11 In whose own image?   175
    Self, nature, supernature and belief

References   186

Index   197

Foreword

I am an editor of a scientific journal, the *British Journal of Psychiatry*, and I aim to publish 'original work in all fields of psychiatry'. My problem, and it is shared by most editors, is that original thinking that is not accompanied by empirical data, either obtained through standard qualitative and quantitative methods, is dismissed as idiosyncratic, odd, speculative or 'preliminary', and the writer is sent back to scurry around for evidence before he or she has the temerity to send the paper in again. Derek Steinberg's book, if shortened into article form (which I acknowledge would be impossible), would certainly come into one of these rejected categories if submitted under our present pressure on space, and in addition to these concerns my referees would suggest that the work is not in 'a field of psychiatry' and therefore not appropriate for the journal. And, of course, as soon as the theme of 'consciousness' is mentioned in good scientific circles, the reaction is the same as that of Stuart Sutherland quoted in this book: 'nothing worth reading has ever been written about it', with the final phrase unsaid, 'and never will be'.

This is a pity, for it is worth remembering that the stimulating and provocative writing in this book was the standard method of scientific discourse from the earliest days of scientific enquiry until less than a hundred years ago. What has changed? The true scientist will answer that we no longer have to wade through pages of long-winded prose and can cut to the quick by reading punchy short articles under tight editorial control. But without Steinberg's type of discourse we would all be the poorer. Here we have an author who is both a polymath and a scholar, who has the courage to incorporate psychology, neurophysiology, psychoanalysis, attachment behaviour, genetics, mathematics, philosophy, evolutionary theory and religion into one volume, and can give good and proper justification for it. I have never been able to understand fully the concept of the unconscious mind introduced by Freud, but Steinberg, by combining discussion of both the unconscious and conscious mind, has given invaluable insights into both.

In one of the early chapters of this book we are treated to the neurophysiological and psychological complexity of a short journey by bus. After reading this account you will be amazed how we get around so successfully. But we are now getting too rigid and organised. All our bus journeys are short ones, the destination has to be clear in advance, the route has to be precise, and we must know the exact journey time. Reading this book is like one of the best of those old mystery tours. We start at the beginning – at least this is familiar – but then we travel through the valleys of metaphor and the peaks of lucid prose, to places we never knew existed, across lands with incredible panoramic views and amazing flora and fauna, have our senses heightened and sharpened, and our intellect strengthened, and finish somewhere apparently unknown but where we still somehow feel at home. After such a journey one can only say, 'Wow!'.

Peter Tyrer FMedSci
Professor of Community Psychiatry
Imperial College, London
July 2006

Preface

This book is about the most remarkable phenomenon in the universe by far, more astonishing than the 'Big Bang', more extraordinary than the origin of life, more remarkable than the development of science, civilisation and the arts. Without Consciousness illuminating the cosmos with thousands of millions of points of light, nothing would be astonishing, extraordinary, remarkable or even of interest. In one way this is a statement of the obvious; yet it takes quite a shift of perspective, emotionally as well as intellectually, to really appreciate that without Consciousness ... nothing. We tend to take it for granted, like gravity, except when in particular circumstances it ceases to be available.

By Consciousness I mean human, reflective, self-aware consciousness, the sense of 'I', that unique individual both the reader and the writer know well, indeed far better than anyone else, however close, and however expert. In most of the recent vast literature on human consciousness this core 'I' at the centre of individual experience seemed to be largely noticeable by its absence, either discussed inadequately, side-stepped or acknowledged (at the close of even some of the most impressive books) as remaining a complete mystery. When I conceived the idea of this book I decided to try to pursue the question of this elusive 'I', even if I had to end up with much the same kind of conclusion.

One assumption with which I began was that, when pressed, most people would have to take the view that *either* the source of the 'I' was supernatural and divine – in other words the soul – *or* it required a biological explanation; and my task in this book was to push biological understanding to the limit. I would be invoking both psychodynamic theory on the one hand and the arts on the other in support of the biological case, on the basis that these too have their biological, evolutionary roots.

Halfway through the book – which became for me a journey of exploration rather than an account of an already formulated story – I found the biological *versus* supernatural thesis wasn't that simple; indeed, like a spacecraft having trouble with the atmosphere, it started losing tiles and other bits and breaking up. This opening note about the book's general drift isn't, of course, the place to sum up the new doubts and new questions that my initial assumptions generated; but the new answers I found myself contemplating, while not so very far from the original starting place and trajectory, did seem to be in a quite different kind of place.

Derek Steinberg
July 2006

About the author

Derek Steinberg has been involved in the arts in one form or another before and throughout his training in medicine and specialisation in psychiatry, and in this book he gives them the prominence they have had in his clinical work and teaching. He trained at the Royal London Hospital, the Park Hospital in Oxford, the National Hospital for Neurology and Neurosurgery, Queen Square, and at the Tavistock Institute and Maudsley and Bethlem Royal Hospitals, where he directed the Adolescent Unit. Despite the Maudsley's admirable eclecticism in psychiatry and neuroscience there remains a deep divide in education and training between the sciences and the humanities in all fields which limits rather than enhances understanding, where academics and practitioners tend to be specialist while the questions they attempt to deal with are generalist. Nowhere is this more the case than in the field of consciousness.

The author teaches nationally and internationally, using arts principles and methods whenever they help. He has published some 60 papers and chapters. *Consciousness Reconnected* is his ninth book, the previous eight following a trajectory from clinical and scientific work towards the arts. He is currently working on an illustrated book about the sculpture, landscape, science and history of the Island of Portland, near where he lives and where he is learning to sculpt. He is a member of the Portland Sculpture and Quarry Trust, and a Trustee of the Bethlem Royal Hospital Arts and History Collection.

Other books by Derek Steinberg

- *Using Child Psychiatry* (1981) Hodder and Stoughton, London.
- *The Clinical Psychiatry of Adolescence: clinical work from a social and developmental perspective* (1983) John Wiley, Chichester.
- *The Adolescent Unit* (1986) John Wiley, Chichester.
- *Basic Adolescent Psychiatry* (1987) Blackwell Science, Oxford (trans. Japanese).
- *Interprofessional Consultation: innovation and imagination in working relationships* (1989) Blackwell Science, Oxford.
- *Letters from the Clinic* (2000) Brunner-Routledge, London.
- *Models for Mental Disorder: conceptual models in psychiatry* (with Peter Tyrer) (4e) (2005) John Wiley, Chichester (trans. German, Japanese, Russian).
- *Complexity in Healthcare and the Language of Consultation* (2005) Radcliffe Publishing, Oxford.

Acknowledgements

It seems to be unusual to acknowledge the authors listed in one's list of references, and yet such is the nature of the subject that I feel warmth and gratitude even to the writers I disagree with, or don't understand. Thinking and writing about consciousness is hard work and sometimes mind-boggling. I feel particular regard for that wide seam of intelligent commentary on mental life to be found outside psychology and the neurosciences, in the arts, poetry and literary criticism.

I am indebted to the teachers and multiple philosophies of the two centres where I received what I think of as my most significant training and experience, the Maudsley and Bethlem Royal Hospital, and the Tavistock Institute. I would not have liked to have known only one of them; this would have felt like having half a brain, though fortunately for psychiatry and psychology there has always been a certain amount of traffic, sometimes covert, between these two great institutions, as between other equivalent centres of the scientific and the intuitive. At the Tavistock, where I was a postgraduate, part-time student for a few years, the time I value most was as a very junior participant in a series of seminars led by Dorothy Heard, Irene Caspari, Denise Taylor, John Bowlby, Anthony Stevens and Colin Parkes, where for me the first seeds of this book were sown, although I found that further plantings were needed in other times and other places. Earlier I had worked and trained at the Park Hospital for Children and the Warneford Hospital in Oxford, where David Taylor and the late Christopher Ounsted might have been surprised, or perhaps might not have been, that some of their highly individualistic and sometimes idiosyncratic perspectives on developmental science and on the necessary connectedness between very different concepts and disciplines flit like phantoms in the following pages.

Beyond the institutions, conversations and in some cases shared teaching about the links and overlaps between the arts and the sciences that I have had with the following friends and colleagues have been particularly important – for good or ill – in shaping this book. The order is very roughly chronological. The late, sadly, Dr Jafar Kareem of the Inter-Cultural Therapy Centre, London, particularly for his inspirational contribution to our discussions on those *other* cultural differences, those between disciplines; Giorgos Polos of the Arts and Therapy Centre and Danai Papadatou of the Faculty of Nursing, Athens; Christiane François of the British Council, Port of

Spain, who helped me liaise with some key people in psychiatry, psychology, teaching and the arts in Trinidad; Professor Jaczek Bomba of the Jiagellonian University, Cracow, for valued discussions about art and psychotherapy; Professor Shozo Aoki of Kawasaki Medical School; Gavin Bird, artist; John Fowles, friend and neighbour, who came so perceptively at psychology and philosophy from the direction – among other things – of geology, history and the particular about people and places, especially introducing me to aspects of Thomas Hardy I'd hardly thought about, and whose extraordinary depth and breadth I think is still being discovered; Ornella Reni, painter and sculptor and worker with psychiatrically troubled people in Como, for conversations about both these aspects of her work which owed nothing to jargon and convention, and for an illuminating meeting on her balcony overlooking the town and lake with her ex-tutor, Professor Ugo Sambruni. This was ably interpreted by Rosemary FitzGibbon, with a thought-provoking conclusion about creativity and madness that one of the most important issues for sanity and consciousness was *responsibility*. Dr Bob Speer, Imperial College astrophysicist and now innovative bookseller of Lyme Regis who, sometimes a little baffled but always intrigued and patient, helped me in my efforts to translate between quantum physics and psychology and back again. Any misunderstandings are mine and due to transmission problems across vast spaces. And particularly John Spencer, a most formative influence who taught me art half a century ago, and with whom I was able to renew acquaintance quite recently and continue some wonderfully disputational conversations. But there were many other conversations with many other people, because whatever the occasion or topic, as many know to their cost, I would sooner or later turn it to the subject of this book. My very special thanks to my wife, Gill, for all her support and secretarial assistance at a more demanding time than is usual, even for the long-suffering spouses of authors.

Thank you, also, to AP Watt Ltd, on behalf of the National Trust for Places of Historic Interest or Natural Beauty, for allowing me to quote from one of Kipling's poems, and to Faber and Faber for permission to refer to the play *The Madness of King George*.

I also want to thank Gillian Nineham and her team at Radcliffe Publishing for a level of responsiveness, helpfulness and efficiency outstanding among publishers.

It may be routine for writers to end such words of thanks by taking responsibility for the mistakes and misunderstandings, but it is something that still needs to be said, and I acknowledge it here.

A short walk around the subject

Something to begin with

What the artist and philosopher Jean Dubuffet (1967) said of art is true also, I think, of that elusive phenomenon human consciousness. *'It does not come and lie down in the beds we make for it. It slips away as soon as its name is uttered: it likes to preserve its incognito. Its best moments are when it forgets its very name.'* Like death or the sun, ideas about the nature of consciousness and self don't reward the gaze of the naked eye. It may even be *necessary*, as I shall explain, for consciousness to be an elusive quarry. Perhaps this is why it remains so, despite the enormous amount of thoughtful and detailed work that has been devoted to the subject. In this book we will try to creep up on it from a number of very different perspectives and, to close the net as it were, try to make connections between them.

Something else

Though I hesitate to distract the reader so early from the knife-edge task of deciding whether this is the book for you, may I draw your attention to something other than these words?

What else do you see before you? The pages, obviously, your hand holding the book, and perhaps a table, or your crossed legs. And just beyond, the room you are in, with this and that here and there, maybe bookshelves, cupboards, lighting, and a window with a view across the street to houses or trees.

Where are these? Well, they will be somewhere with familiarity, an address and the other attributes of place. I have no doubt that you could find your way around them, for example to go to a shelf and pick out, say, a dictionary, and then find your way back to your chair and this page. Now, while I can't know where you are as you read this, I do know that what you are looking at is all inside the back of your brain and represented – no one knows quite how – as an image a few millimetres across and upside down. You might as well be sitting in the dark and observing the scene through a virtual reality helmet. The material room really is there, in a grey sort of way (our brains do the colouring in), but the image you work with is, unfortunately, where I said it is; I say unfortunately because extraordinary and far-reaching though the process is, many people including myself find the notion a little unsettling. And it is more than just a picture. It is not only a holographic image, but one loaded with meaning and value. So were you to cross the room to get that dictionary, you would do so by stepping into a three-dimensional set of your own making, projected onto the outside world from that tiny scene mediated somehow in and through the occipital cortex at the back of your brain. Clearly it is important to get the scene right, and most of us most of the time do seem to manage it. We will return to this and another example later.

Meanwhile, where, then, is the room you're looking at? Out there or in your head?

One response is 'both', but speaking for myself I still find that leaves us with a bit of a philosophical conundrum about that room we can walk around in.

I won't dwell on it further for now, but will make two points about it which represent something of what is to come. First, we will never get anywhere in exploring the subject of consciousness if we take any-thing – like one's self in that room – for granted.

Consciousness, as we shall see, works by being taken for granted, and to stand a chance of glimpsing what it's all about we have to find a way of going behind the scenes without losing our grip on the very consciousness which is our sole instrument for exploration.

Second, if we accept for the moment that what we perceive is both inside and outside at the same time – interacting in a sense, but inter-acting so intimately and at such speed that they, or it, is in effect in both places at the same time (as some of those mysterious particles in quantum physics seem to manage) – then we have a circular model of A leading to B, and B almost instantaneously back to A again.

There is a third point to have in mind throughout what follows. We operate, as I will argue, from an evolutionary and developmental perspective, at three main levels, all at the same time. How we are now, at this moment, depends on (a) about a thousand million years of evolution from primitive cell to contemporary human being, (b) on our individual development in our lifetime from conception to this moment, in other words our personality and predispositions to date, and (c) how we feel about, understand and respond to immediate stimuli, events and relationships. These three levels or phases, discussed again later, have quite different origins but are interactive, in that what we are born with (our genetic inheritance) helps shape what we make of ourselves and our environment as we develop, and what we make of ourselves and our environment influences what we make of each day's myriad experiences, events and relationships.

I, consciousness, self, and soul

By consciousness I mean self-consciousness; not 'shyness', of course, but consciousness of self, the inner and ultimate 'I'. Just about all definitions of consciousness are tautological, in other words defining self-consciousness in terms of itself (e.g. 'self-awareness'). In one sense this is unsatisfactory, but it also provides us with a clue, and the first step in that clue is, again, the circular nature of the phenomenon we are pursuing. We will come back to this point, several times. A persisting problem with defining consciousness is that however industriously we try to define 'I-ness' in a complete and watertight way, there always seems to be another 'I' standing one step back, as if involved, interested, but 'outside the frame'. This is described, sometimes despairingly, as the 'law of infinite regression'; rather like pursuing a rainbow – it is always further away. Again, a rainbow is both in the sky and in your head at the same time: a crowd may contemplate a rainbow, but in optical terms each individual in the crowd has one of their own.

While referring primarily to human self-consciousness, most people would assume that other animals are in a sense conscious. My own assumption is that all the way up the animal ladder – through woodlice to spiders, ants, bees and so on, about which more later – the obvious consciousness of the world around them that these creatures possess is best described as something between responsiveness and awareness; even an intruder detector 'senses' someone entering its range of detection, or a spider is 'aware' of a fly caught in its web, but how similar or different the burglar alarm is from the spider's internal machinery for detection and response (inherited, of course) isn't easy to say. I don't believe that most animals are conscious in that special self-aware sense of themselves as individuals which we possess; not even, unfortunately, the most charming, intelligent and responsive of cats, dogs and horses. Regarding the higher primates, however, and the mysterious dolphins: no one knows, although their use of planning and tools may suggest consciousness of a kind approaching our own.

As to soul: the problem here is that the word tends to be used in a religious and supernatural sense, and as commonly thus used makes all kinds of assumptions. However, if we may postpone discussion of the religious and the supernatural until later, and for the purposes of what leads up to it, I will identify 'soul' with the ultimate 'I' at the core of the person.

Stepping at some point onto the moving carousel

'Nothing can come of nothing', as the fourteenth-century proverb says, anticipating the law of the conservation of energy. I would like to introduce the reader to the most fundamental of the many conceptual models I will be introducing in this book as a peg, or rather an ever-circling energy-transforming platform of pegs, to hang things onto. The cover illustration of this book, the carousel ridden by Mnemosyne, mother of all the muses (of whom a little more later), hung on the wall of my room for some time before I realised its relevance to what I was working on. Was it an unconscious stimulus? Or did I like it because of ideas already taking shape on the back-burners of the mind? Such questions are all part of the particular complexity and circularity I want to describe.

Living systems operate in cycles, not in straight lines. This concept is interesting at the moment – by which I mean the latter part of the twentieth century to the present – in seeming brand new and even a little eccentric at least as far as much applied science and technology is concerned, for example in much of medicine and psychiatry (Steinberg 2005) and yet should surely become common sense. The difference between linear models and circular models and the systems theory that supports them is discussed on pages 37–9. But for the purposes of this introductory framework, let us imagine a child in a fairground spotting a turning carousel.

To jump onto the carousel takes energy. The idea of springing onto it came out of the blue – her mind had been on other things. I don't know how much energy it takes to run alongside an accelerating roundabout and clamber safely aboard, but suppose it is pretty substantial. Does that mean that the completely new idea itself already contained the energy to alert and interest this young person and produce some kind of physiological summation of intention and muscular activity? Presumably yes, because nothing can come of nothing. Suppose the idea comes to me to ask you to cross the room to shift a heavy piece of furniture; something I imagine you hadn't thought of. Suppose you do it. How does the energy involved track through the squiggles of printed ink on the page from my sudden and bizarre idea to your muscular activity? Because I don't imagine you had thought it up yourself. Firing nerve cells involve energy-consuming chemical processes, and provide the physiological machinery for what seems to begin with an entirely new and abstract (and imaginary or even illusory, if you like) act of will. *Can* a 'new idea' be energy-free? Presumably not, however 'out of the blue' and fleeting.

I referred earlier to the mystery of the 'I' that seems always to be one step back from any theories of 'I' which an 'I' can propose. This and the conundrum of the origin of an act of the will have both been considered as representing the philosophical puzzle of infinite regress, for example that any voluntary act of will must by definition be itself initiated by a *preceding* act of will, or it wouldn't be voluntary (Ryle 1949; Dunne 1958).

I think the problem of how a new idea can appear, generate intention and serious activity and then impacts on the world (or the furniture) lessens somewhat if we think in terms of cycles. Something like a predisposition or potential to take action, locked up in physiology and internal imagery, is already there and releasable. Circularity may help with the 'in the brain or in the room?' conundrum. One answer – mine – is both; no need to fix on one locus or the other, although that is how we often tend, unthinkingly, to think.

And what lies behind motivation is complicated. To jump on the roundabout takes confidence ... or something; but it could also take wilful disobedience of parental instructions, or of a warning sign on the side of the carousel, or of a shout from its operator. This will have its own history in that child's development and family. It could be related to whatever, socially or chemically, underlies risk-taking, or conceivably even a behaviour or hyperactivity disorder. It could relate to issues of intelligence, foresight and judgement and mood. Moreover, fairground attractions, warning signs and the authority (acknowledged or not) of the carousel's operator are all significant cultural perceptions, as is all the myth, glamour and enticement of the fairground. I have gone on about this wide and variegated range of reality and perception because Consciousness seems incomplete without it.

Such phenomena represent the socio-cultural feedback system which contributes to the self-conscious state, whatever else is influential as well. Thus, the child could be justifiably confident of her aims and athleticism because her parents and other key people nurtured, encouraged and recognised this quality in her and reinforce it appropriately. Being treated as confident and competent helps confidence and competence and feeds into self-identity. Alternatively, a child in a family which is neglectful for any number of possible reasons could be at risk in that fairground. Being treated as someone who can do what they like regardless can – *via* the exchange of subtle social signals within the family – lead not to confidence but to lowered self-esteem and even self-negligence. And suppose the child was in an essentially normal family but had a condition that affected her mood and judgement that day? Or in a family that couldn't stop her being high on drugs? Will, memory, behavioural repertoire, relationships, the situation, the cultural setting, all the fun of the fair and taking risks all contribute.

Take any action or state of consciousness, trivial or elaborate, transient or enduring, and it is not difficult to see it as enmeshed in a complex network of neural, psychological, social and cultural connections. And they are all as homeostatic (i.e. dynamic: ever-changing in the interests of stability which itself is adaptive and able to change with circumstances) as the chemistry that keeps our neurological systems stable and our bodily fluids life-supporting; indeed marine-like, carried with us by those of our remote fishy and then amphibian ancestors who successfully (or we wouldn't be here now) moved onto dry land; which was even more risky, whatever its attractions, than climbing onto a moving roundabout. Our nervous system grew from and through such origins too. In what follows I will argue that the 'I' is forged from all of these processes and all this history.

These are the most basic and simplistic of the concepts underlying consciousness as I will discuss them in the following chapters. Not consciousness as merely something buzzing between the ears, to be explored by peering into the head with ever more sophisticated devices; but consciousness as something brain-rooted, certainly, but dependent on the outside world as well as the inside world and the infinite, dynamic complexity of both. You will notice that I have slipped evolution in too. The reader may be aware, if he or she wasn't already, that to invoke evolution in psychosocial matters can provoke as much distress and even rage in some social scientists as among creationists; perhaps more so. This bizarre and unholy development in the politics and emotions of contemporary science is mentioned again on page 17; but, be warned, treading on such feelings could cost jobs, exam passes and more: do see Rose and Rose (2000) and Segerstrale (2001) for a comprehensive review of the debate.

Now this is all very complicated. I have even invoked political considerations in the previous few lines. However, I suggest that this is the kind of complexity that needs to be grasped to form viable concepts and possible hypotheses of how minds work and generate consciousness, rather than by by-passing these biological, psychological and social areas. This has involved burying the subject in highly abstruse notions of mathematics and information technology, attempted by many authorities on the subject (critically reviewed by John Searle, 1997), in which consciousness seems conceptualised as a property of a very elaborate and complicated computer – some kind of lap top, but on our shoulders.

Where, then, in terms of using the model I have outlined, to start the cycle? Obviously, at any point: biological, neurobiological, psychological, philosophical, social or cultural. What matters for the proper study of consciousness is not to dismiss the other parts of the cycle. And yet this, remarkably, is how the subject is generally approached.

The rest of the fairground

The state of the study of consciousness at the beginning of the twenty-first century involves, appropriately, a degree of bafflement and controversy, particularly over the question of the core nature or even existence of something called Self – i.e. you and me. Carter (2002), in her comprehensive, up-to-date and accessible review of the field, found herself gratified that her publisher allowed her to say not only that she didn't know the secret of consciousness, but that she didn't think anyone else did either. As recently as 1995 Sutherland, in compiling his *International Dictionary of Psychology*, was able to say that 'Consciousness is a fascinating but elusive phenomenon: it is impossible to specify what it is, what it does and why it evolved. Nothing worth reading has been written about it' (Sutherland 1995). I think this is a little unjust, although Güzeldere (1998) thought Sutherland's words worth quoting respectfully in the introduction to his and his co-editors' monumental, multi-author anthology of the subject (Block *et al.* 1998). Most authorities (Popper and Eccles 1977; Penrose 1990; Dennett 1991; Edelman 1992; Crick 1994; Chalmers

1996; Searle 1997; Greenfield 1998; Damasio 2000; Malik 2000; Carter 2002; Humphrey 2002; LeDoux 2002; McCrone 1990 among others) acknowledge the mystery of self-awareness at the heart of the subject. Dennett (1991), who is as familiar as anyone with the conceptual, commonsensical and other problems of consciousness, describes it as the last surviving mystery: 'Consciousness stands alone today as a topic that often leaves even the most sophisticated thinkers tongue-tied and confused'. He contrasts consciousness with just about any other subject of enquiry – for unlike any other phenomenon, 'any particular case of consciousness seems to have a favoured or privileged observer, whose access to the phenomenon is entirely unlike, and better than, anyone else's, no matter what apparatus they may have' (Dennett 1991). He means, of course, you and me. In a sense the exploration of consciousness is the ultimate task, for every other phenomenon, from photosynthesis to gravity, can be explored using our conscious minds; to explore consciousness *with* consciousness is difficult, to put it mildly, especially if, as many including Dennett suggest, consciousness is a phenomenon created ('spun') by the mind, and has the qualities of an illusion about it. No wonder some conclude that conceptualising the 'I' cannot be done.

However, all this will not put us off, because while some think sophisticated mathematics or machinery will themselves give us the answer by delving ever-deeper into the brain and computer-generated imagery, cells and chemistry in search of the soul, the ultimate I, this will never be achieved; rather, there is something to be done by standing well back instead, and using the extraordinary, I-generating equipment we all carry around between our ears.

Now, our brains and minds (which I will regard as one) are capricious, curious, and much given to fantasy and narrative, deception, self-deception and being deceived, in other words to creativity and invention – frequently of an astonishingly high order. This emergent thinking and behaviour is creative, sometimes hyperactive, often eccentric and occasionally mad. All this sounds more like art than science. Beginning with the notion that comes again and again from the serious scientific and philosophical literature on the subject, *that self-aware consciousness has some of the qualities of an illusion*, I am going to see whether those not ordinarily invited to take part in scientific discourse, for example artists, poets, film-makers and other illusionists, theologians and people with particular kinds of psychological troubles, can help illuminate the subject. If self-awareness is indeed one of the greatest illusions of all time, what we can learn from biochemists, neuroanatomists and data-crunchers is unlikely to be enough. Pursuing the metaphor of the Great Illusion, we also need the illusionists: artists, poets, writers, producers, directors, lighting engineers, cameramen and set designers – all sorts of shapers and illuminators of our worlds; and an attentive audience: one evolved to take an interest. And magicians too.

But in case any reader is alarmed at the direction being taken, don't suppose that consciousness would be any the less for being illusory. The whole of art and literature is an elaborate kaleidoscopic illusion, is it not, and none the less real for that? What are for example London, Venice, Europe, America, Africa, 'The East', a beautiful sunset, a rainbow, the ceiling of the Sistine Chapel, the Mona Lisa, your favourite writing, books, films and plays, in fact just about anything you can think of, including history, economics and even 'hard' currency, even gold and diamonds, but enormously elaborate and finely crafted consensual illusions, albeit rooted in realities? Even what one may most like or dislike about relationships and acquaintances may be illusory, and none the worse for that. Past and future are necessary illusions. They exist only in the neural present (itself a few milliseconds behind in 'real time') as imaginative constructions between memory and a concept of past time on the one hand, and anticipation and a concept of future time on the other. We exist in a creative world of virtual reality, as will be demonstrated and discussed in terms of both the oldest and the newest philosophy.

My purpose is not simply to assert that self-consciousness is 'merely' smoke and mirrors, as though something else were 'more' real, but to affirm the importance of the subjective reality of illusions, and to see if, and how, they may be connected with the somewhat harder data and theories of neuroscience, psychology, social science and biology; which have more than their share of subjectivity too.

Federico Fellini, the great film director, coined the phrase 'real dreams' for an autobiographical film (Fellini 1987). As implied in the Preface of this book, we would do well not to allow ourselves to be entrapped by Manichean (and essentially linear) concepts of dualism, where everything is categorised into A or B, good or bad, black or white, etc. This too is an illusion (pragmatically and in evolutionary terms a convenient one), driven by the compulsively categorising (and in this sense prejudging) brain with its physical structure reflected in the dynamics of the human psyche (*see* pp. 12,15). Is a dream, or a film for that matter, real or illusory? Obviously, it has the qualities of both categories. A metaphor I will increasingly elaborate in this book, therefore, is consciousness not as circuits in a computerised box, but as a performance – starring, directed by and with script, scenery and locations – by one's self, with the circuits being between brain, self and the world outside.

What else is on show? Top of the bill, of course, neuroscience. The roots of consciousness are in the physical brain, even if, as I will be suggesting, what grows from these roots as consciousness is far more than that. The findings and views of neurophysiologists and brain chemists, as well as clinical neurologists, constitute the subject's solid foundation. The brain is emphatically *not* like a computer (*see* pp. 14, 49 and John Searle 1997); I would go further and say it is quite unlike a computer. For a start it creatively, imaginatively and unpredictably programmes itself, all the time coping with uncertainty, ambiguities and self-contradiction. It is disobedient and deceptive, and driven by emotion as well as cognition.

The broad subject of biology is inseparable from neuroscience in importance here, particulary evolutionary biology and the science of the genes. But these also overlap with sociobiology – social biology and animal behaviour (Wilson 1979, 1992). This field also overlaps with psychology, and the subject which I will propose as central to the theme of what follows is Bowlby's attachment theory (e.g. Bowlby 1969, 1973, 1979), which began as the science and psychology of how young primates (human and animal) grow and develop by relating to those looking after them (Tinbergen 1951, 1953), but has implications for the whole life-span.

Attachment theory in turn involves the fields of family, group and social relationships. It also relates to the cognitive and emotional development of the individual child and adult, and the particular aspect I intend to make the special focus of attachment theory, for the purposes of this book, is the process by which the developing human being constructs for himself or herself an elaborate inner imagery of the outside world; and, I will add, of the world within as well. This, in turn, is related to the kind of imaginative work and fantasy with which psychodynamic theory, developed by Sigmund Freud and his followers, is concerned.

Where do the building bricks of this image construction come from, bearing in mind the earlier aphorism that 'nothing can come of nothing'? First, from our memory, both from earlier experience and from perceptions of a few milliseconds ago. Second (and I think it deserves a second category because it represents a move from memory as cognition to memory as affect-laden), the 'colouring-in' of a perception by real or fantasised past experience and emotionally-laden anticipations about just about anyone and anything.

Feelings and cognitions are dynamically generated, ideas and emotions feeding each other in yet another cycle. In a reasonably competent person there is a sustainable, realistic final common path, to use the classic neurophysiological term (Sherrington, 1906), but managing it is like being an acrobat on a tightrope on a see-saw on shifting sands. Fortunately most of us are 'good-enough' acrobats (*see* p. 82).

Psychodynamic theories and primitive imagery

What is in the mind's eye can be sophisticated and elaborate, and pretty definite, but other categories of inner imagery are more primal, and represent the developing mind's efforts to make inner representations of feelings about perceptions at a stage (developmentally) or a level (now) when there are neither words to use for them nor experiences to relate them to. They are powerful 'feeling complexes' rather than visual images, but because they are powerful and universal, being rooted in instincts from a time when we were *all* instinct, they have a kind of familiarity about them. They become distilled into the self-description, self-justification, folklore and mythology of the human race as 'human nature'. They are fundamental to Freudian theory and that of his followers and, needless to say, remain subjects for dispute. Brown (1961) provides an excellent short, clear summary of the main psychoanalytic schools, and for those interested I recommend his account as an introduction, Hinshelwood's first-rate discussion of Kleinian theory (1994), Stafford-Clark's *What Freud Really Said* (1983) and the introductory book by Storr (1989), and also the master himself, Freud (1954), who was a considerable writer whatever conclusions are drawn about his theories. CG Jung (Brooke, 1991; Storr, 1998) is in an important category of his own.

At this point I will simply try to convey the essence of the kind of inner imagery psychoanalytic theory is about. It is also referred to as fantasy, but in terms of qualities and levels of consciousness I feel this is perhaps too definite and cognitive a term for either phenomenon. Like dreams, imagery and fantasy may seem vivid and clear until you try to pin them down into words and pictures, as writers and artists know only too well. Melanie Klein's theory, for example, assumes that the first stirrings of an emerging mind exist in, indeed consist of, chaos: a kind of emergent raw awareness with no clear boundary between the emerging sense of self and the emerging sense of what's outside the self. It is, I think, rather like the state of the amoeba as discussed later (*see* p. 54), drawn towards what evolution determines is good for it (e.g. nutrition), and away from the bad (e.g. toxins), yet without awareness; but the emerging mind I am discussing has the advantage, or burden, of a super-added dawning consciousness.

Given the rudiments of a mind that starts from here, the early developing mind (we are talking weeks here) begins to become aware of the desirable and the disastrous – somewhat like a sensate amoeba, but with someone looking after it – 'good' things (like being held, comfort, being fed) and 'bad' things (like being put down, being uncomfortable, not being fed). Thus out of the inchoate primal awareness, which I suppose is something like being in a dream, or very intoxicated, an idea grows that it (I think it is too early to say more than 'it' – the Freudian word is 'Id') is the recipient of good things and bad; but more than merely good and bad, rather extreme, primitive, unmodulated feelings of helplessness, hatred and rage on the one hand, or intense love and gratitude on the other. Brown (1961) put it well by saying the emerging child, or mind, finds itself in a world peopled by Gods and Demons. Klein describes this period as a paranoid stage of development. The experience called 'good' becomes identified with a figure who keeps reappearing, classically the child's mother, which may be the first time inchoate feelings begin to take some shape. But then there is the 'disappearing' mother who puts the child down and leaves the room. As the early mind puts two and two together it finds that the object of its vast gratitude (in Kleinian language, the 'good object') is one and the same as the 'bad object'. Negotiation of the discovery that the loved and hated 'objects' are one and the same is regarded in Kleinian theory as an important formative stage and ushers in the foundations of uncertainty, doubt, reflection, reappraisal and the loss of basic certainties. Melanie Klein regarded this as a maturational step from the 'paranoid stage' of development to the 'depressive stage', with depression in this sense regarded as something with its positive aspects, and ushering in tolerance of ambiguity instead of total reliance on illusory black-and-white certainties. She was describing an infantile, developmental stage; but psychoanalysts, traffic wardens and airline cabin crew know that no one is too grown up not to regress to paranoid rage in certain circumstances.

All this is speculative, naturally, but I think those who find it plausible, if not completely convincing, do so because it seems reflected in adult lives too and also in the monsters, good fairies, witches and wizards in every kind of nursery rhyme and folk story. Booker (2004), in an informative work that spans psychology, particularly Jungian theory, and literature, points out that taking all the tales the human race tells itself, from mythology to novels, there are only a limited number of basic plots, largely based on the hero's actual or metaphorical journey – the quest – to achieve a great goal, with terrible difficulties to overcome with the powers of goodness and badness helping and hindering, sometimes untidily, all the way. Lives and novels, 'good' ones and 'bad', have much in common.

I have described what I will call 'proto-imagery', i.e. yet to become explicit as language develops and in narrative, literature and art, at a little length because I think it is no less plausible than much of the more mechanistic and mathematical material in many books on Consciousness, and I will predict that it will be more enduring, and more useful, in our attempts to conceive Consciousness. Psychoanalysis and the arts generally seem to me to represent a crucial connection in the net of consciousness between (a) animal instincts and how they evolve, (b) the developing mind and how it begins to make sense of itself, (c) the stories the human race tells itself, again to make sense of itself and its surroundings, and (d) the beginnings not only of creativity but of an imperative drive towards creativity – to make sense of what would otherwise be chaos. The whole is an adaptive, imperative impulse born of curiosity, memory and apprehension; the latter in more than one sense, meaning perception, uneasiness or both. Burnshaw (1982) has described this process with poetry as the focus and biology as representing its ultimate roots.

Archetypal imagery

The student must beware, because the above kind of thinking and literature is controversial, indeed practically taboo in some scientific and psychological circles; psychodynamic thinking in particular tends to be regarded as counter-intuitive by those suspicious of intuition. Archetypal psychology is even more so. CG Jung (e.g. Stevens 1990; Storr 1998) appeared to maintain that the kind of imagery described above was actually *inherited*; that it was innate, coming with the genes. For many this was worse than nonsense – it was heretical, an anathema. I will discuss archetypal imagery – Gods and Demons, Mother Figures, Father Figures, Wizards, Witches and Monsters – later, because they have a key part to play in my account of the emergence of the conscious self. For the moment I will draw attention to a great misunderstanding, one perhaps due to some of Jung's own accounts of his theory: as Jung eventually himself affirmed, these inherited phenomena were emphatically *not* inherited images, but the predisposition, in the nuts and bolts of the physical nervous system, *to be capable of forming such imagery*. Thus, as we shall see in Chapter 9 which reviews neurological contributions to the Consciousness debate, a notion dismissed even up to the present as so much mysticism is brought right up to date in the language of genetics and neuroscience (though characteristically without mentioning Jung or the word 'archetype').

The story so far, and a twist in the tale

First, my general theme. Consciousness is never going to be grasped by an appeal to philosophy alone – although this constitutes a significant part of the literature – nor to neuroscience alone, which makes up an even greater part. Understanding what neurones do is necessary but not sufficient for comprehending consciousness. The idea that computer science can take the subject forward will prove a particular blind alley; I agree with Searle (1997) that those who understand the world through the medium of information technology seem overly emotionally committed to force consciousness and mental life generally into its mould. My own view is that computer science is merely the latest (and also transient) conceptual model for making sense of the world of the mind, just as magic, gods, demons, spiritualism, hydraulics and geology (in psychoanalysis) and more recently mathematics and quantum physics have been. Like its predecessors, computer science will leave a handful of concepts about consciousness which are interesting or occasionally useful. As to mathematical models (e.g. Hofstadter 1979; Hofstadter and Dennett 1981; Penrose 1990, 1994), perhaps these brilliantly occupy other worlds entirely. We will be returning to them.

'Consciousness' as a term by itself is short of meaning, except, possibly, denoting linkage to the *unconscious*. 'Consciousness *by*' and 'consciousness *of*' begins the process of giving the category some connection with what we experience. (Perhaps Consciousness could usefully be designated as '-C-' rather as carbon atoms are in organic chemistry.) We shall see that this step – giving consciousness a kind of connection to the phenomena and processes described – will also contribute to both a definition and description of consciousness.

If I am setting aside neural anatomy, physiology and computer science as by themselves insufficient for comprehending consciousness – I do not set aside philosophy, from the classical writings of the last few thousand years to writers like Humphrey (1984, 2002) – what am I adding to the argument?

With regard to the role of neuroscience, not only can I not see any case for consciousness surviving that does not have its roots in physiochemical brain function, but some of the neurological accounts of the basics of consciousness are impressive. The problem is, once again, our over-determinedly categorising human brain, which neatly encourages us to side-step the task of seeing *all* that is involved. Why on earth *should* consciousness be primarily understood only in terms of neuronal circuitry? Despite the meticulous, beautifully argued cases for a neural origin for consciousness (for example by Edelman 1987, 1989, 1992, 1995, 2005) one might as well (to use the metaphor to which I keep returning) try to grasp the world of film by peering into a DVD machine, a cinema projector, or by sitting in a meeting of cinema industry accountants, or scriptwriters, or advertising executives, for that matter. Why should the subject of Consciousness *not* be as widely diverse as the cinema; or as zoology is for that matter? Zoologists don't argue that an account of the animal world is complete by describing the reptilian evolution of scales or eggs, habitat-selection, or the chemistry of haemoglobin or digestion in isolation from each other.

To approach even the beginnings of what consciousness may be, we do need neuroscience and philosophy, but we also need to take account of:

(a) that which actually completes our conscious minds – our experience of the world outside: the contents of consciousness. I will argue that these don't 'fill' consciousness; they *make and shape it*, set its boundaries

(b) theories of the unconscious mind and the external influences of social psychology

(c) that which the mind *does* – the whole of its creativity and innovation: in the broadest sense, for good or ill, its productivity of ideas, arts and artefacts.

These three categories are remarkable for their almost complete absence in the colossal literature on Consciousness of the last 30 years or so.

*

So much for my explanation of the approach of this book – what Victorian authors, with studious vanity, in an elaborate preface, used to call 'the author's apology for his book'. But the twist in the tale is *why* we should be so narrow and super-specialised in our approach to the subject. My hypothesis is that the bigger the topic the more we trust in the depth of understanding at the cost of breadth, a point I have made elsewhere (e.g. in Steinberg 2005; Tyrer and Steinberg 2005). The cost is considerable. And the final *twist* in the twist is that this curious motivation, or at least so far as consciousness is concerned, is to an extent explicable by the *nature* of consciousness; that it is subjective and elusive, and perhaps has to be to work. Thus, we use ever finer pins, when we really need to cast a wide net.

Uncomfortable bedfellows: the view from under the sheet

I hope the relevance to the study of Consciousness of biology, different aspects of psychology (e.g. memory, perception, mental imagery, social relationships, psychodynamic theory), neuroscience and the mind's creative capacity will be reasonably obvious. However, looking for connections between such fields is the exception rather than the rule. Indeed, you have only to read a little widely to see that many of the protagonists of one field will readily dismiss others which they either don't, or don't want, to know about. Not only will the geneticist or neuroscientist not lie down, figuratively speaking, with the social scientist, who in turn will not even speak to a social biologist or evolutionary psychologist, but within psychodynamic theory, that apparently most open-minded of fields, the Freudian may well have little time for the Jungian, and the Jungian for the Kleinian. As to artists and poets having anything to do with the debate – perish the thought. Later, and even worse, I am going to bring in theologists too.

I have known a biological psychiatrist get hot under the collar about Freud – 'that obscene scribbler' – and a social scientist dismiss him simply as 'a liar', while, more politely, a lecturer in the philosophy of literature in his liberal intellectual uniform of smart jacket and jeans, after a longish conversation which had seemed to represent a meeting of minds, explained that he was 'very uncomfortable' about my interest in evolutionary psychology. Social scientists with an interest in the mind are to be found who regard biologically-orientated psychiatrists and psychologists, and indeed biologically-minded human biologists too, as 'fascists' (see, for example, Rose and Rose (2000), Segerstrale (2001)). As to what evolutionary biologists think of theologists coming onto their territory, and vice versa, or whether many behavioural psychologists would think art theorists, poets or novelists could throw any light on the mind, we are then well up in the heights of the Tower of Babel – which is the subject of Chapter 3.

Does it matter? Doesn't science proceed by argument and refutation? Yes; but some sort of dialogue is required first, and an attempt to see what the other field's contribution might be, rather than the prejudicial and often quite emotional jumping to negative conclusions which is quite common among otherwise serious-minded super-specialists. The subject is then deprived of the broad-based approach it needs; and, worse, such attitudes become institutionalised so that from appointments committees to journal editors, from academic departments to examinations, a subject which can only be understood holistically is rigidly compartmentalised. We arrive at the situation where a senior academic in one area necessary to the subject is likely to know less about another necessary area than an undergraduate.

To reiterate the twist in the tale – a double twist: the way our brains are made, that is the way we think and the way our limitations and primitive emotions (e.g. territorial defences) lead us to construct our institutions, academic organisations and other enterprises, is only half the problem. Recalling Dubuffet's quotation about art at the start of this chapter, I will be arguing that consciousness *works* by being elusive and to an extent illusory; the difficulty of seeing the whole picture – including the difficulties we make for ourselves intellectually, academically and largely irrationally – may be in part related to the way the conscious mind works towards maintaining its own integrity. In books that pioneered the philosophy of biology and mind, Gregory Bateson (1973, 1979) made the point that the enormous difficulty we have in grasping the nature of consciousness is itself a key part of the phenomenon. To keep our sanity – so it seems – we *need* to break the subject down into digestible bits and pieces; to try to be, say, scientist or artist, biologist or psychoanalyst, or geneticist or social scientist. More generally speaking, to allow for both the objective and the subjective is often regarded as idiosyncratic and incorrect. That way, it is implied, lies madness. My own view is that that way lies sanity, and an opportunity to grasp the nature of consciousness.

Again, a recurring theme in this book: narratives (like the Babel story) and belief systems are intimately related, and likely to convey in different ways the message 'don't meddle in things you aren't supposed to understand'. This could be not only for traditional reasons of folk philosophy, but because tribal leaders and story-tellers of one sort or another (remember human minds made up these tales) might well have thought that knowing or even questioning too much might be bad for you as well as subversive, and best left to the High Priests. I don't think that the prevailing institutionalised and largely academic censure on too much intercourse between (for example) art and science, science and religion, or genetics and social science is all that different – to which our contemporary High Priests will protest that in these cases they really *are* right; but then High Priests always do.

The rest of the book

Chapter 1 has been a preliminary ramble about the subject and how I propose to deal with it. I mentioned attachment theory not as a 'unifying theory' (beware of unifying theories of large topics) but as a system which provides an open framework for a number of evolutionary, behavioural, psychodynamic and socio-cultural concepts that need to be brought together if we are to understand the nature and origin of human consciousness. I argue, with Gregory Bateson, that the difficulties inherent in the subject are actually *part of the phenomenon* and therefore where we should seek some of the answers; this is because consciousness and the elaboration of an 'I' represents something of a creative performance which does not lend itself to be readily understood by peeping behind the scenes. I hope I have made it clear that invoking creativity, imagination and illusion in the production of a phenomenon does not diminish it. Rather the reverse.

Chapter 2 is an attempt to describe and define the subject and some of the other key words in the title and subtitle. The essence of this chapter, however, taking up the case that some very different kinds of fields need to be explored, is that different kinds of thinking are needed too. Neural, mathematical, cybernetic, cognitive psychological, psychodynamic, biological or theological thinking alone will not do; each is too limited for the subject. We may prefer or even need to be specialist, and owe much intellectual and pragmatic achievement to our tendency to categorise, but the breadth, depth and dynamic fluidity of consciousness suggests a generalist, holistic set of processes in its operations.

Chapter 3 takes up the theme of institutional confusion and lack of imagination not (or at least not only) as a gripe, but to argue that in the interests of nurturing and maintaining consciousness the brain sets traps and diversions to divide and divert those who would try to get to the bottom of it. How? By elaborating cautionary folklore: 'I wouldn't go there if I were you', sort of thing; or stories about forbidden fruit and the penalties of embracing the Tree of Knowledge. Such stories, like those of the Tower of Babel or the Garden of Eden, are hallowed, institutionalised, inscribed on scrolls, leather-bound, made into films and quite likely carved in stone; but they nonetheless originate in human brains, not in the clouds of Parnassus or other mysterious peaks. But, as we shall see in Chapter 11, this is not to diminish them. Rather the opposite: they are part of human psychology.

Chapter 4 outlines the feasibility of the sense of Self emerging from its origins in a few chemicals in the primeval slime, as life's first environment is engagingly known. While the rest of the book is an account of disconnected parts and ways of joining them up, this chapter is an attempt at a continuous narrative, based on the connections living forms have with each other in addition to their obvious differences.

Chapter 5 is an account of attachment theory, and the pivotal role I have given it as a meeting place for evolution, psychodynamic theories and the emergence in the human mind of patterns of imagery which are vivid, remembered, expressed and adaptive. Evolutionary theory often relies on one or other kind of material hothouse, typically dramatic in nature and effect, for example the blazing nuclear reactor of the sun, condensing vapours on the grandest of scales, sliding tectonic plates, burgeoning forests, asteroids crashing into the earth creating vast dust storms, each great scene kicking evolution forward via changes brought about in climate or territory. In attachment theory I suggest another sort of hothouse: that of the hypersensitive, feeling, empathic, manipulative, fantasising, scheming, deceptive, self-deceptive mind – an emotional hothouse in which all kinds of strange things grew during millions of years and which became our conscious and unconscious minds, involving the emergence of ever more elaborate fantasy and imagery, sometimes rewarding, sometimes horrific, of who we are, where we are and of the significance for good or ill of other people.

Chapter 6 is about what blooms and thrives in this hothouse and, staying with the principle that living systems are better represented by cycles than straight lines, how that which grows from the hothouse – narrative, myth, language, philosophy, social constructs and all of the arts – feeds consciousness too.

Chapter 7 takes one of these cycles: how some of the imagery which evolutionary and ethological processes produce becomes incorporated in the evolution and ethology of the human species, thus providing a possible scientific basis for CG Jung's still controversial notion of the archetypes of the collective unconscious. It is then argued how this can be a route for perceptive capacities getting into the gene pool of the species, and thereby contributing tangentially to that other highly controversial, indeed largely abandoned, notion of Lamarck's, the inheritance of experience of the outside world. The evidence that individuals can pass such experience 'back to' and onward in their genes is scanty and dubious at present, although discovery is full of surprises. But species *can* shape themselves to social as well as physical environments.

Chapter 8 is about art, in its broadest sense, and is a reminder that the physical brain and its internal psycho-physiological workings, for all its astonishing power and capacity, is only part of the story. Art and artefact of every sort comes from the mind and feeds back into it. Just as the brain has its key areas, neuronal tracts and synapses, the culture that the brain feeds and in turn feeds from also has its pivotal, mind-shaping influences, its points of focus, those things that have fed into that reciprocity I have identified between mind development and cultural development. Continuing with the theme of making connections, I will give examples of the impact of art and developments in the arts on the developing mind and vice versa. I will suggest that the arts occupy a crucial intermediary zone, neither wholly subjective nor wholly objective; art, in fact, as both play area and crucible for the development of human self-consciousness and self identity.

Chapter 9 is a tentative construction of a model for the self-conscious mind, with the brain as the physical substrate for an elaborate cycle of perception, self-perception and the processing of internal imagery, culminating in the emergence of the *I*. The chapter represents the neuropsychological component of a reciprocity between inner and outer worlds, between the primarily neural and the primarily cultural; a 'central processing unit' where the brain integrates the inner psychic worlds and the outer social-cultural world and produces a Self.

Chapter 10, a short clinical interval, discusses whether identifying consciousness as something beyond the merely 'mental' might throw any new light on aspects of clinical and therapeutic practice in mental health.

Chapter 11 was difficult enough to write, still less to try to summarise here. It is an attempt to face some of the mysterious gaps and loose ends that invariably result from exploring human consciousness; to see whether we can go some way to understanding them – not tying them up – by seeing if they occupy a place which is neither wholly natural nor supernatural. It is an exploration of whether there may be something beyond monism and dualism (*see* p. 91). Triadism?

Finally, I thought I would attempt a summary of the essence of the whole story in a (longish) sentence – something for the writer if not the reader to hang onto. It is this. Biological reflexes, instincts and simple representations of the environment, surviving because they were shaped by evolution, are then amplified and augmented by powerful feelings, memories and imagery when the evolutionary necessity in primates for personal attachment brings into the equation social as well as biological imperatives, and – because they are crucial for survival – these feelings, memories and imagery become established in the species' nervous system as archetypes which straddle brain and culture.

2

Consciousness disconnected

The title, some definitions, and ways of thinking about consciousness

> *I cannot totally grasp all that I am. Thus the mind is not large enough to contain itself: but how can there be any part of itself that is not in itself?*
>
> (St Augustine AD 354–430, *Confessions* 1961)

Consciousness and the sense of self

Again, there has been not one Big Bang, but three, and of these the most extraordinary by far is the emergence of Consciousness. Consciousness, that is, in the human sense, awareness not only of a range of stimuli, sensations and perceptions such as animals show, but a subjective sense of personal identity, of the self, at the centre of individual existence. This is what this book is about. Later, when we review what others have made of the subject, we will see that the issue of the core self has often been evaded one way or another, sometimes left out of the argument, and sometimes described as the ultimate mystery, possibly one beyond all objective explanation. I have a certain regard for this latter conclusion because for all that it is ultimately unsatisfactory, it does indicate the size of the question.

One of the aims of this book is to try to find ways of conceptualising consciousness and our sense of self, albeit that it is near-indescribable, because we are attempting to grasp the nature of our self-consciousness with our self-consciousness, something akin to lifting ourselves off the ground by our bootstraps. Within an infinity of cosmic time and dark, insensate space, each individual's sense of personal identity flares into infinitesimally brief moments of existence and then fade again – like a shooting star – as far as we know forever; yet in that split nanomoment of cosmic time with nothingness on either side, each human being becomes so much individually, in terms of memories, anticipations and relationships, and within their role, small or large, contributing to whole cultures and civilisations. It is as if next to nothing becomes everything, and this represents an extraordinary biological and psychological event and a phenomenal philosophical puzzle: even poets, and I include the writers of hymns, parables and prayers, struggle to describe the astonishing nature of this phenomenon adequately. Among the many strands of motivation for this book is my impression that many true scientists and artists seem ever more awestruck, more struck by wonder and strangeness and inspired by what they continue to find in nature, while so many leaders and followers of the 'official' religions seem to take it all very much as a routine. It is as if attributing creation to God – admittedly with enormous respect – sets neatly to one side the capacity and need to be astounded and dumbstruck by it all; which is, I think, the more appropriate reaction. Nevertheless, one must seek the words to describe it if one can, and here, to my mind, the best artists and poets lead the field.

Consciousness not quite defined

Definition means a precise description, one that delineates the subject and distinguishes it from everything else. I haven't yet seen one which works for consciousness, since most rely on one or other version of 'self-awareness', which is tautological and therefore not quite satisfactory. But later I will argue that, for reasons I will explain, tautology may be just what is needed.

Damasio (2000), whose account of consciousness from a neurophysiological perspective is, I think, among the more important, begins somewhat reluctantly with the dictionary definition that it is an organism's awareness of its own self and surroundings. One feels for him, and many others – because all this kind of definition does is deftly substitute the word 'awareness' for consciousness (i.e. what is consciousness? Answer: consciousness).

Dennett's notion of an infinity of kinds of sentience, to which ambiguous term he adds the more precise concept of responsiveness, is helpful, but doesn't quite get us to human self-consciousness, and he introduces the disappointing notion that as we work down the scale from our own experience of consciousness, and up the scale from primitive biological responsiveness, contact is missed 'like ships that pass in the night' (Dennett 1991, 1997). Later I will dispute this in pursuit of my own account of what human consciousness may represent.

Greenfield, who starts out from the perspective of primarily neuro-physiology and biochemistry, describes consciousness as 'the inside-the-skin sensation', which is a start, but leaves out the recipient of the sensation. She too is troubled by Dennett's notion that the closer we come to trying to explain first-person consciousness the more irrel-evant it seems (Greenfield 1998). Like Dennett, she draws our atten-tion to different kinds of consciousness, which is important, and in an earlier book (Greenfield 1997) provides a neurochemical model through which gradations of feeling, which she places close to the nature of human consciousness, are biochemically modulated and fine-tuned. The perspectives of both authors, the one more philo-sophical and metaphorical, the other neurochemical and neuroana-tomical, provide a mutually consistent matrix composed of physical brain processes and abstract thinking processes which will be useful later. In Carter's wide-ranging review (2002) she says of the field's output of some 30 000 papers, '99 per cent talk only about the "easy" peripheral issues: how consciousness is generated; what it contains; who or what has it ...', not the subject's 'hard' problem of what it *is*.

In another key contribution to the literature, Block and colleagues (1998) raise the stakes with a near thousand-pager, with some 40 authors and 50 chapters, in one of which Goldman (1998) observes that our attempts to define consciousness are largely through 'unrevealing synonyms', *but this does not necessarily show that anything is amiss* (my italics). Again, I think the topic's very elusiveness is the nub to understanding and, ultimately, defining it. As said earlier, Güzeldere (1998) opens this comprehensive and authoritative review of the field with the acknowledgement in his Introduction that consciousness largely evades definition, and with Stuart Sutherland's gritty con-clusion (1995) that it 'is a fascinating but elusive phenomenon ... Nothing worth reading has been written about it'.

So there we are. But *courage mes braves*: as I suggest throughout this book, the very difficulty of defining and conceptualising core self-consciousness, and the tautologies we resort to in making the attempt, is an important part of the answer.

Other words in the title

But back to the basics. By *neuroscience* I mean the study of the hard-ware of the mind: the brain and its neural structure, function and biochemistry, and also its developmental history in the individual and its evolution in the species. Mind and brain are so interconnected, especially as argued here, that rather than resort to using 'mind/brain' as is sometimes adopted, I prefer to use the terms separately, but always with the implication that where one goes, the other cannot be far behind. When the distinction matters for the argument I will try to be consistent in referring to the neural or physical brain on the one hand, and the psyche as the concept that goes beyond the physical brain. No doubt I will be inconsistent at times.

By *psychology* I refer primarily to psychodynamic (or 'depth') psychology and to social psychology. ('Depth' psychology is a term I have noticed only in one or two places, for example as the title of an excellent book by Dieter Wyss (1966)). I mention it to denote a whole group of psychological schools of the unconscious mind, for example Freudian psychoanalysis, Jungian analytical psychology, Kleinian psychology, and all kinds of anthropological, philosophical and existential schools, all to do with that aspect of the mind which combines some qualities of subjectivity and narrative consciousness, and yet is either just out of reach of the conscious mind, or so 'beneath the surface' that its existence and contents are simply inferred.

On the subject of things unknown or at least not obvious that affect the way we think, feel and behave, I am going to include in this category another sort of 'unconscious', but one whose origin is social, from without, rather than from within: the way in which social and cultural phenomena and processes influence or even determine attitudes, feelings and motivation. It is what political radicals refer to when they talk of 'raising awareness' (e.g. of disguised authority, or economic forces) and is the equivalent, though in another direction, to what dynamic psychologists call 'insight'.

By *the arts*, I mean the creative arts generally (drawing, painting, sculpture, music, drama, dance and literature) and beyond these the humanities in general. However, the common denominator I have in mind here is the process of making images and using words and symbols, particularly in myth, poetry and metaphor, in music, drama and movement. Much of this comes together in the cinema, and I will give a special place to film because it provides a whole range of analogies for the mind, from the technology of the equipment to the ideas, scripts, drama, landscapes, scenery, creativity and *dramatis personae* involved. Its metaphors, as I will show, straddle both the 'software' and the 'hardware' of the mind, conscious and unconscious intentions and motivations, and conscious and unconscious perceptions; and, above all, imagery and narrative on a grand scale, which is what the mind is involved in. All this is a very broad remit, and necessarily so, my argument being that what the mind *experiences and does* throws as much light on consciousness as what it *is*. This breadth is, I believe, very broadly in line with what Dawkins (1976) and Blackmore (1999) mean by 'memes': replicated ideas and artefacts, subject to a kind of adaptation and evolution. Elsewhere I agree with those who dispute the assumption that the mind is largely a super-powerful computer. However, a metaphor from computer technology is useful where the role of the arts is concerned, in that the archetypal psychology to which I give a central role in consciousness provides the means for neural strategies learned in biological adaptation to become evolved into the hard-wiring of the brain and then by socio-cultural evolution into the permanent structure of the socio-cultural environment – the software. Straddling brain and culture, it is one of the most important connections to be made.

By 'art' I don't mean only the 'official' or recognised arts, but the capacity in individuals for imagination and for making something to do with living skills out of what was in the imagination, as well as the capacity to notice and even appreciate the aesthetic. In other words, a kind of proto-art, a potential for art, which I give a pivotal role in the mind–culture cycle, each feeding the other, and from which 'big Art', the recognised art of galleries, libraries, theatres, film and concert halls, is simply a fallout. Institutional art is important, but it is not the raw stuff. I do want to emphasise this broader pro-cultural penumbra to art: the names, roles, status, activities, addresses and origins we attribute to ourselves, the dates and times we construct around our lives (even strapping them to our wrists), the things we hang on our walls, our fashions and decorations, these and a myriad of other small arts and artefacts, all mirror and help cement our identity. In this context, Big Art is only a by-product of this characteristic of the human race, albeit with a transcendental grandeur of its own.

The same applies to the artist, in which group I include every sort of writer, poet, story-teller and mythologist, whether culturally recognised or not. Artists, in the broadest sense of the word, and that deep-rooted within humanity which appreciates the arts, represent a whole other world of the human mind on the subject of mind and consciousness; yet it is largely excluded from the neurobiological debate, and appears only patchily and in rather specialised forms even in the subjective, intuitive world of psychoanalysis, where Freud seemed to regard art, like religion, as a kind of neurosis.

The recent *scientific* literature on consciousness, as mentioned earlier, is large, influential and growing, and largely rooted in neurobiology. There is another, longer established literature on the *philosophy* of the nature of consciousness, and it overlaps with work on spirituality; I am thinking of a whole ocean of classic writing, from the foundation works of all the major religions through the poets and philosophers to the classics of fiction; and since it isn't feasible to list their extent I will pick out a few names to illustrate those who have a particular place: in religion and philosophy Plato, Meister Eckhart on Christian Mysticism, Baruch Spinoza, William James, Karl Jaspers; the writings and philosophy of Hinduism and Sufism, which is mystical Islam, and the Buddha, the Bible, the great myths of the world, and Moses de Leon, the Spanish kabbalist believed to have compiled the Zohar. As far as my title is concerned, I have conflated philosophical writings with the arts and humanities, to distinguish them from objective or quasi-objective science.

In literature generally, I would mention Shakespeare, Goethe, Marcel Proust and Thomas Hardy as among those who made special and now classical contributions to psychology. In an essay on a much wider circle of writers (including Henry James, the psychologist William James' brother), David Lodge (2002) describes what are in effect the narrative threads on the loom of consciousness, the neuropsychological weft going the other way to complete the weaving process. I would take this argument even further, and say that everything that minds produce, all the 'art', from works of genius through the everyday (especially the everyday) to transient rubbish, is part of the picture of consciousness; that the emerging mind (emerging in evolution as well as in each of us in our individual lives) weaves around itself a kind of localised mini-culture, a psychic cocoon or nest, which builds and maintains the personality, a range of states of mind and how we relate to people, places and things, so that there is a crucial reciprocity between creativity (including creating junk) and self which stitches our sense of ourselves together. Thus in private ruminations, or knowing the classics, or watching TV, or functioning among family and friends, man makes art and arts make man. This is going to be a key theme in this book and will emerge more fully later. But for the moment I mention all this because to grasp the nature of the conscious mind, we need to try to get to grips with the contents of consciousness and its dual source, from within and from without; and what the active image-laden, fantasising, communicating brain constantly contributes to both sources. To return again to the question (*see* pp. 1–2):

is the mind in the brain or outside? One might as well ask whether human respiration is all about the oxygen in the atmosphere or the haemoglobin in the blood. The answer is in the reciprocity.

Inner and outer reality

By 'imagery', then, do I mean inner imagery or outer imagery? I wish there were a clearer answer to that, other than to appeal again to reciprocity. It is a baffling conundrum, perhaps best left alone after a brief and respectful acknowledgement. But it is not to be glossed over, being an important strand in the mystery of Self. Richard Gregory (for example 1987, 1997, 2005) has worked and written extensively and particularly accessibly on this near-baffling issue.

I would like to give as an example of my own the following situation, not unlike that given at the beginning of the book. You are waiting for a bus, and at risk of being late for something important. A big red bus appears in the distance. It takes some time before you can read its number, and twice, frustratingly, it stops at another bus stop, and then at the traffic lights. As it comes closer you see it is your bus, and as it stops you jump aboard and buy a ticket. I fear we are describing the late lamented Routemaster here, as was recently dismissed from London streets. As it lurches off and around the corner you manage to scramble up and around the spiral staircase, clutching a couple of bags as well as the somewhat greasy-feeling rails and poles that help you on your way; and you get to a seat at the front where you can contemplate wherever you are heading and whether you will make it on time.

In doing this you have demonstrated the extraordinary nature of the virtual reality helmet balanced on our neck and shoulders. What you have seen and acted upon – the distant and approaching bus, the successful jumping aboard, the leap up and round the stairs – has been perceived upside down and with left–right reversal scattered across a few millimetres of brain inside the back of your head. And that is only the least of it, in terms of the complexity of the visual pathways. Jumping on the bus is a considerable neuropsychological and acrobatic feat. The distinguished neurologist McDonald Critchley, at a lecture at Queen Square – the Institute of Neurology in London – once commented on the extraordinary ability of the brain to lock the outside world into place, in perceptual terms, as we walk about in it. You only have to turn your head to observe this phenomenon – and this represents only one feat among the many the brain performs without us realising it, to sustain the contact with the outside world we take for granted. The disabling condition of true clinical vertigo (which is not 'dizziness', nor fear of heights) conveys what happens when this complex mechanism falters. There seem even to be separate visual pathways for seeing the bus and climbing aboard it.

So where does that leave the 'outside world'? It's there, few have any doubt about that (some philosophers have demurred, for example George Berkeley (1685–1753)), but the material world is not necessarily as it seems. For a start the bus isn't 'red' or any other colour until its image is being processed between the retina and the brain; so what about size, position, feel, smell and so on? I will not try to resolve this business here, but want to remind the reader about where we are going, so to speak. Somehow, miraculously I would say, we create perceptions as a result of complex incoming stimuli from a world outside our virtual reality helmet and space suit, from which we then project outwardly (onto what?), and having achieved this quite amazing creative act, we step into this world and live our lives in it – every second of every day. The mundane act of catching the bus is connected by a whole three-dimensional web of other connections, both without, in the 'real', external world, (including bus routes and other topographic maps) *and* including the inner worlds of other people which we observe, interpret and react to; and *within*, connecting with roots in the conscious and unconscious levels of our minds too. It makes a difference, does it not, if an old friend, or for that matter someone we don't like the look of, climbs aboard 'our' virtual reality bus, as does the significance of our journey, and whether we are late or early.

I would not call this fragment of imagery, projection and action a unit or building brick of consciousness – that would be premature – but it does represent a kind of prototype unit of existence and awareness. It will do for now, and we will return to it from time to time and use it to build more elaborate models. But at this stage we are thinking about the mere basics of structure and function – anatomy and physiology, and quite elementary cognitive and dynamic psychology.

To anticipate some of the narrative to come, I will try again to sum up the framework of the rest of the book as briefly as I can: it is about how consciousness and the sense of self can emerge from a reciprocal relationship between a developing brain and nervous system and the developing culture the brain spins outside it, like a vast,

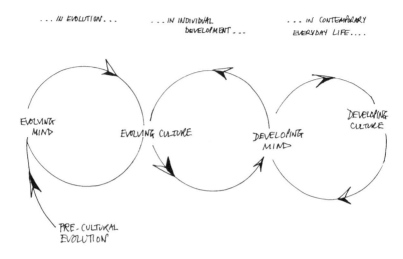

Figure 2.1

multi-dimensional tapestry (*see* Figure 2.1). And how vast, if you add recollections (real and imagined), anticipations, predictions, hopes, fears and fantasies to this bigger picture. Hence St Augustine's plea (Pine-Coffin 1961) at the start of this chapter; and the thought that however big the universe, the mind is bigger. It is said that the number of possible permutations of connections between the brain's neurones – one hundred thousand million of them – *each* connecting with 1000 to 10 000 other cells exceeds the probable number of atoms in the universe. I don't know if this is accurate but it seems unreasonable to dispute that frequently quoted order of magnitude.

Moving from what the brain is to what the brain–culture interaction does, and taking just one small measure of brain productivity, it is worth considering by way of a light interval how many different books, fiction and non-fiction, have been written and could *ever* be written, through the agency of the human mind, using the alphabetical letters of a grid no more than five by five – most languages are composed of similar numbers of letters. Is the answer infinity? (*See* Figure 2.2.)

This reciprocity between the developing mind within and the developing culture outside (and catching buses and bus routes are as much part of culture as art, science and relationships), all this and the feeling-laden and fantasy-laden imagery which mediates it, is

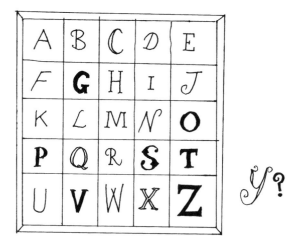

Figure 2.2

crucial to the argument I am putting forward in this book. It is why the model of consciousness as proposed here is not one obtained by merely peering into the contents of the skull and wondering what is happening in there. That would be like – is indeed like – trying to grasp the nature of the Internet by taking a lap-top apart. Yet much of the explanation of consciousness proceeds in this way.

A question about imagery: imagery and its observer – 'Io'

A further thought about the internal image, since I have given it a central place – you cannot have an image without an observer; but nor can you have, I believe, a phenomenon of so 'pure' and finely distilled a consciousness that it isn't illuminated by anything: it is hard to imagine a kind of 'awareness', presumably consisting of pure thought, yet *sans* sight, *sans* sound, *sans* smell, *sans* taste, *sans* feeling, *sans* proprioception (position sense), *sans* every kind of symbolism experienced or recalled, indeed *sans* everything. Conversely I doubt whether without some kind of retained, potentially memorable imagery, however nebulous and however symbolic (for example like a word on the tip of the tongue and searched for, perhaps unsuccessfully, or in the vaguest memory of a dream, just out of reach), there can be, phenomenologically, consciousness. There seems to be, therefore, a crucial duality at the heart of human self-consciousness: an image of some sort, and an observer of some sort. Without the one, there cannot be the other: something seen, or apprehended, and something doing the seeing and the apprehending. I am therefore suggesting that 'consciousness', the noun used for convenience, might be better thought of as a transitive verb, 'consciousness by' and 'consciousness of'; thereby implying its participation in an active circuit. I will identify this tentative contribution to the model of consciousness, when it seems helpful, as 'Io'. (Io, like Mnemosyne, Goddess of Memory and mother of all the creative muses, was a mistress of Zeus.)

This implies that the term consciousness, while convenient, is misleading: pure 'Consciousness' is a kind of anti-oxymoron: I suspect it cannot stand by itself. For a word that has inspired such a huge literature by itself it is remarkably short of meaning, which perhaps makes sense of Daniel Dennett's impatience with it (Dennett 1969; Searle 1997). As suggested on page 15, I think that you can only have 'Consciousness' *by* and *of*. Thus no consciousness without imagery, and no imagery without an observer. So we are looking for a two-headed beast, here in the conceptual jungle, or in the head. Later we will see that these thoughts about the nature of Consciousness (a term I will hang onto for convenience) bear a relation to the arguments made neurophysiologically by Damasio (2000) and Edelman (e.g. 1989) and perhaps by Dennett (1969, 1991, 1997) to the extent that I can follow his philosophical argument and his debate with his critics. But also, more controversially, by Jaynes (1976), who involved *hallucinations* in his account of consciousness.

Despite my probing the notion of 'no consciousness without imagery', where does that leave hallucinations, dreams and the unconscious? And especially dreams: do they represent imagery that generates a consciousness, vaguely recalled, in the sleeper?

Meanwhile, despite being an archetypal non-mathematician, I cannot help wondering if we have the beginnings of an equation, or at least equivalence, here: that $Io = -C-$.

Some other concepts needed en route

I have already indicated the ways in which we need to think, if we are to stand any chance of constructing a comprehensive image or model of the mind. Some are commonsensical, others perhaps less comfortable to go along with. As pointed out earlier several of them, or rather their proponents, may appear to be strange bedfellows.

1 *Acceptance of different kinds of language for different kinds of form and function*. Perhaps the greatest distinction is between descriptive language (like neurone, or an item of behaviour) and metaphor (like 'levels' of psychological organisation, or elaborate metaphors like 'Oedipal conflict'). Some terms stand for both the literal and the metaphorical, e.g. exploratory behaviour, or projection. The famous image in Stanley Kubrick's film *2001* of an ape throwing a bone spinning into the sky, and which, turning against the sky, became a space station, represented at least three kinds of projectile: flung bone, a projected idea across half a million years, as well as a highly creative metaphor for progress. Language and symbolism are key phenomena throughout and they link psychology and the arts, encompassing neural evolution and function, psychological development, multiple levels and implications of meaning and much of culture. Narrative, the telling of stories – to and about oneself as well as to and about others – is part of the fabric of brain and psychological function on the one hand and social life and mythology on the other.

2 Respect for *mythology* is related to this, and is important. It is curious that even when myth is treated by its detractors as synonymous with untruth, it is as if, paradoxically, 'mythology' is regarded as representing another kind of historical and classical world of reality altogether, somewhere between ancient dusty libraries and Hollywood, and to do with manufactured nonsense about Gods and Goddesses, with no connection with the brain at all. Yet myths are the products of the real, live brains of real, live people much like ourselves and our contemporary leaders, elites and opinion-formers, who told each other yarns much as we do now, and for rather equivalent reasons of instruction, warning, persuasion and the identification and defence of actual and metaphorical territory, and for much the same political and ideological reasons. Dismissing such stories as irrelevant to the science of the mind is as irrational as dismissing, for example, clinical symptoms.

On a political note, I would question whether the determination of tyrants, activists and other ideologists has as much to do with domination as ordinarily understood as it has with a need to shape the consensus about the sanity or common sense that I related to early human evolution (*see* pp. 35, 45–7, 100, 129). Because, however much you try to define a delusion in a clinically watertight way, it breaks up on the rocks of 'what most people think', and in the end is culturally determined. The emotional drive behind even the most rational of political and other intellectual persuasion is, I suggest, a struggle for authority about what shall be the prevailing 'normal thinking', rather than for the intellectual or moral high ground. This too is part of human mythology, and is not soft stuff; I agree with Lewis Wolpert, evolutionary biologist and wood-touching atheist, who argues for the evolutionary necessity of conviction (Wolpert 2006). We are descended from the kinds of ancestors who were convinced there was food on the other side of the river or that a particular kind of berry was safe to eat or that the gods would back a particular line of action, though obviously not from those who tried to walk across the water or were otherwise wrong. But one way or the other, for us, conviction carried the day, and the genes.

3 Being open to *intuitive* as well as *objective* information is necessary, because both represent ways of understanding different aspects of mental functioning. A psychoanalyst may be averse to trying to measure what he or she is achieving with a client, seeing it as beyond measurement, for example how a fragment of a dream or fantasy vaguely *feels* from moment to moment, or how one image of someone conflicts with other images. Yet it is true that even the most elusive of subjective feelings could be measured at least as absent (0) or present (1), and no doubt a behavioural psychologist could devise ways of measuring the way fragments of observable behaviour correlate with records of changing feelings, e.g. of warmth or coolness between therapist and client. It could be done, but attempts have often failed because of the gulf, emotionally and conceptually, and again perhaps politically, between the two kinds of observer.

4 Hence *complexity*: a willingness to see, first, that explanations of consciousness are unlikely to be simple, and, second, that they are likely to be most authentically represented by a range of conceptual models. For example a state of anxiety, if we are to describe it fully, would need to be represented by the following: biochemical changes, physiological changes, various kinds of behavioural changes from slight facial expression to complex behaviour like running and hiding, by conscious thoughts about what is causing anxiety and what might relieve it, by the kinds (subjective) and patterns (objective) of relationships which provoke degrees of anxiety or conversely relieve it by degrees, by misunderstanding

and misinformation, and also by images in the mind, some clear, some vague, some of real things, some of imagined things, and some more or less shadowy or unconscious, and all concerning what is feared, *and* of what may help; and so on. And by the various cultural *meanings* of the term. All of which is also a way of describing levels of psychic and neurophysiological organisation at any given instant.

5   This (point 4) represents a kind of *cross-sectional* here-and-now look at what is going on at any given moment (*see* Figure 2.3), from the (metaphorical) depths of the unconscious and the actual chemistry going on at synapses (the nerve connections) all the way to how one or more people are overtly behaving, i.e. from the chemical to the cultural. But we need also to think in terms of causation and undercurrents (*see* Figure 2.4):

(a)   *Temporally* – how they fluctuate over time, from milliseconds (= right now) to years.

(b)   *Developmentally* – that is, changes during growth from child-hood to maturity.

(c)   *Ethologically* – which is about the causes, development, func-tion and evolution of thinking, feeling and behaviour, over many millions of years. As said earlier, (c) influences (b) which in turn influences (a) – all the time.

   When someone becomes enraged about someone parked illicitly on his drive, it represents a very ancient anger indeed. (Or even when a behaviourist finds a psychoanalyst parked on his territory, or a sociologist discovers a social biologist on the shortlist for a job in his department).

(d)   In terms of *relationships* between pairs and small and large groups.

(e)   In terms of the *wider subculture and culture*, as discussed in later chapters, particularly 6 and 8. Moreover, it is not fixed (not 'carved in stone', as they say when alluding to mythology) but constantly changing, and in the mind–cultural reciprocity already referred to, each individual influences, and in turn is influenced by, the prevailing socio-cultural setting to a varied extent. This is a big subject, and as full of controversy, fudged thinking and argument as any other discussion of conscious-ness. This isn't surprising when one considers the human energy and ingenuity devoted to battles over what is the 'normal' (or 'correct', when authoritarianism is confident enough to ex-pose itself) way to perceive, feel, think and behave; what is

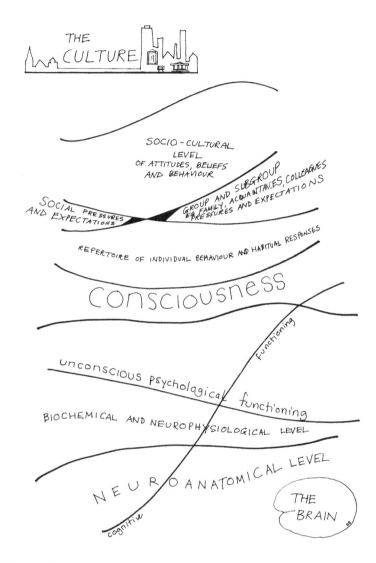

Figure 2.3

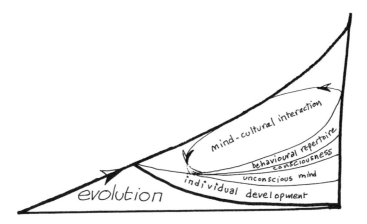

Figure 2.4

socially and politically acceptable or 'best', and what is academically acceptable, is also in constant flux. All this is based
on ideas and feelings and is largely emotional, subjective and
illusory, but wars are fought (and stopped) over such arguments. Millions are killed for them, i.e. individual offending
consciousnesses wiped out, and, in the end, the sword does
seem more potent than the pen; but at the other end it is the
idea, the mythology of a culture or subculture, which drives
the sword, or the car bomb. Subjective emotion may seem soft
stuff, but has impact.

Any given cluster of feeling, attitude and behaviour about
matters small and large from how to style appearance and
behave in public to staying alive is worth trying to understand
in evolutionary terms, within the lifetime of the individual in
developmental terms, within the 'present state' at any given
time, and within personal, group and social relationships. It is
at least as vast, complex, dynamic and 'busy' as the neurochemistry of brain cells, and this should not be surprising, as
each mirrors the other.

6 *Systemically*, that is to say recognising how things, especially in
living systems, affect each other in networks, cycles and spirals
(Von Bertalanffy 1968); spirals because a few turns of a cycle may,
by incorporating new information outside the initially closed
cycle, move it to another level. Thus, internally self-reinforcing and
cycling feelings may jump to a new level with maturation, experience

and circumstances. A simple example is the confident, socially skilled person (brought up that way) who as a result elicits positive reinforcement from others and becomes a still more confident person (*see* Figures 2.5 and 2.6). Circularity describes and explains such processes better than linearity (*see* Figure 2.7).

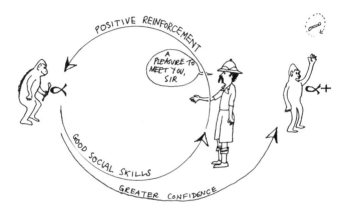

Figure 2.5

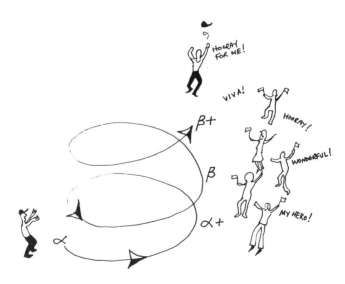

Figure 2.6 ... with one turn of the reinforcing cycle, our hero feels more confident in that relationship. By carrying this into other relationships, the circle begins to spiral, and he becomes a different person, less dependent on external reinforcement

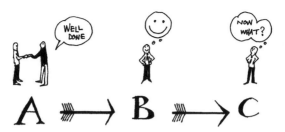

Figure 2.7   The limitations of linearity

7   *Dynamically*, which is to say that how someone feels or responds represents an outcome, transient or persisting, of the interaction of any or probably all of the above levels.

8   We also need to think *philosophically*, because of the difficult concepts involved in describing and attempting to grasp the nature of reality, distinctions between *why* and *how* things happen, the meaning of the term 'unconscious', or where exactly the mind is located. Philosophical questions include the careful and critical use of language; how we think affects how we use words, and how we use words affects how we think (see Heil 1998; Bolton and Hill 1996).

However, it isn't only a matter of conflict over ideas and words. Misconceptions can creep in by accident; for example, even in the most exalted scientific circles one can hear evolution described in terms of 'the animal developing a different skin, or jaw, or reproductive system, in order to ...' etc. Or, from a distinguished scientist, 'the distance from the sun is finely adjusted – not so close that we are burned, nor yet so far that the rays from the sun would be too dim to allow the chemical reactions upon which life depends'. Finely adjusted? By whom? It is not that the earth is finely adjusted to us; we are here, after an absolute holocaust of lost living or potentially living things, because our ancestors were a peculiar minority who could manage and thrive within an extraordinarily narrow band of heat and oxygen. The world isn't finely adjusted to us – we are finely adjusted to it, and at an unimaginable cost in terms of 'failed' life forms. As Richard Dawkins vividly puts it, ancestors are rare, descendants are common (1998) and 'we are going to die, and that make us the lucky ones'.

9 It is important, as said earlier, not to take anything for granted, as if 'given' or 'just there' without seeking further explanation. We might for example observe that man is a social animal, to use a common cliché, without appreciating that exploring *why* man is a social animal says something about the nature of mental life and consciousness. That which we 'have' – our basic ways of seeing, thinking, relating to each other and knowing who and where we are – seems 'natural', but that is because step by step it all has its origins and development in brain and mind. It is not 'given' that a parent cares for a child, or that the child even notices the parent. These things evolve largely by trial and error, and are present in Dawkins' 'lucky ones'. To explore how something as fundamental as consciousness developed, we must begin at the very beginning and track forwards, which is why I chose to start with the cell, for example the amoeba.

The same is true of every other aspect of evolution: our vision, more brain function than eye function alone, is a particular response, one that worked, in the type of light that existed in the flux of cosmic physics and in the environment our ancestors were in. All this may seem a rather pedantic argument, but in attempting to clarify the elusive subtleties of psychological behaviour, cause and effect, how particular capacities began and developed, such abstractions as the meaning of words become relevant to the nature of what we are examining. Take, for example, 'attractiveness' – which will emerge in our discussion later on. I hope it is obvious that beauty does indeed lie in the eye of the beholder; we may categorise a human face as beautiful, but the word is objectively meaningless in relation to a layer of more or less hairy skin stretched across bones and teeth and containing various holes, through two of which moist coloured spheres peer out. 'It' is not beautiful in any absolute aesthetic sense, though we may say it is literally attractive; *we* attribute to *it* our feelings that it is beautiful. This doesn't diminish the status of beauty; it is just a reminder of its source and nature. The philosopher Alfred North Whitehead (1947) said that we – our brains – and not the nightingale should be congratulated for the beauty of its song. Whitehead called what we experienced of the song an example of a prehension, a perception coloured both by the perception of the stimulus (the song) and by a feeling tone associated with the perception – a subject–object relationship which he regarded as fundamental to the structure of experience. On page 12 I introduced the Kleinian notion of the child beginning to divide its world into 'good' or 'bad'. It is not however that simple. The child divides the world, certainly, and these primitive divisions into a kind of acceptance and a kind of rejection (the amoeba, once more, this time with feeling) *becomes* the basis for our cultural sense of 'good' and 'bad'. Like evolutionary arguments, like attractiveness, all such things need to be seen not as taken for granted and naturally 'given', but as things which, given time, worked for us and made us. In studying life, psychology and consciousness, one of the most valuable instruments is the retrospectroscope; we need to read things *backwards* from how they turned out for us. Evolutionary success is not pre-ordained. That which worked is judged successful, beautiful, ideal, and we evaluate and shape ourselves and our world accordingly.

10 Since we are dealing with realities, we need to look at the politics of intellectual life too; this also influences what is or is not recorded, acknowledged, debated, or even noticed. The way our minds work at all the different tasks we undertake divides people into different sorts of thinkers, and they become drawn to particular kinds of work, teaching and subjects. This is where some of the greatest difficulties happen in trying to integrate the study of consciousness. The highly focused, mathematical man or woman who favours precision and objectivity might read poetry or enjoy art in their spare time, but might well be surprised or dismissive at the prospect of impressionistic and subjective people like artists, poets and novelists, let alone theologians, having anything to contribute to comprehending consciousness.

11 Finally, about neuronal speed and activity and another great indefinable, Time. Everything about the normally functioning mind seems rather quiet and still within, and this surely affects our concept of brain and thought. The brain seems as silent and still as a phrenological head or brain slices under the microscope; there is the quietness of the consulting room or laboratory, of the images in the viewing room of the brain scanner, or the data on the computer screen as the cognitive scientist pores over it. The image I have of the brain however is of constant and frenetic activity at a multitude of levels, like a vast, teeming city – but speeded up. Sherrington (1906) again on the brain: 'this buzzing loom'.

Tools for the trip

After all this relatively balanced discussion, I hope, about ways of thinking about Consciousness, here are two assertions. They are contrived to act as tools, templates or orienteering gadgets (for they have the multiple capacity of a Swiss Army knife) to carry the argument along.

1 First, the crucial importance of *words*. Letters are the visible signs of the atoms of human consciousness, like the track of a particle in quantum physics; words are the molecules they form and everything from phrases to whole narratives and books represent its chemistry. Did you know, by the way, that a book is called a *tome* because it is sliced, cut up, into pages? An atom (*a-tomic*) was thought for a long time to be incapable of further splitting. Playing with words is also something we will keep coming back to because metaphors act as psychic catalysts. With this in mind, I would like to suggest the metaphorical 'device' in Figure 2.8 as an example of a prototype space/time/consciousness probe for the elaboration of meaning into words: at the centre, the actual *word* itself, the look of it and how it sounds; attached, above, the *meanings of the word*, hanging somewhere between, as we have seen, what the individual's mind makes of it, and what the outside world – the hearer, and the wider culture – makes of it. And below, the way the word becomes embedded, as it must be, in neuroanatomy, neurophysiology, the unconscious and evolution: that aspect with its physical roots in mind, brain and voice; and that aspect of it hard-wired into the brain by evolution. Every time a word lands, that is docks via eye or ear or fingertip, there is a small burst into meaning and the neural–cultural link is established once again.

2 Then there are the shifting sands on which the further complexities of meaning and metaphor rest (*see* p. 44). On page 37 I referred to an aetiological model of the way each bit of behaviour may be considered at several interacting levels – how they are in the *immediate* situation, how they have *predisposed* the individual to react by virtue of his or her personality development to that moment, and how *evolution* contributed to the foundations for both. These are *not* fixed; hence the sliding wheels (*see* Figure 2.9). Thus, how an agitated passenger in a plane or at a check-in desk feels and behaves will depend on how mature he is able to be, which will be influenced by (a) the skill of the crew member, and

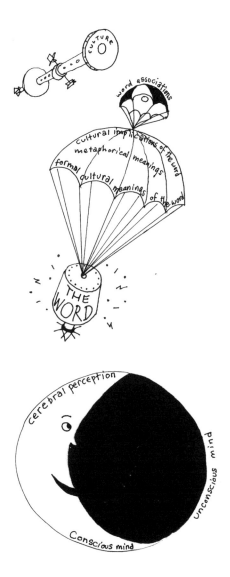

Figure 2.8

(b) how close his general repertoire of social skills takes him to behaving like an ape. This is a fluid (sometimes alcoholic), dynamic situation: a skilled flight attendant, nurse, police officer, waiter, anybody, can usher someone back from infantile rage and ape status – sometimes. Thus, this conceptual model of the state of consciousness at any given moment operates in the *present*, (a) straddling behaviour/mind/predisposition, and (b) is partially explained chronologically by current mood and social skills, by a few decades of development, and by a million years of evolution. 'Slippage' back is known in dynamic psychology as regression.

Thus the image on which we base our self-image and our making something of the external world and acting in it depends on, among other things, what we project out into the world and onto situations, things and people, and regression may happen back to how things might have been handled in earlier personal or evolutionary times. (In Richmal Crompton's William stories the unappeasable Violet Elizabeth Bott would threaten to 'scream and scream until I make myself sick'. Both represent alternative primitive or immature ways of connecting with and handling reality.)

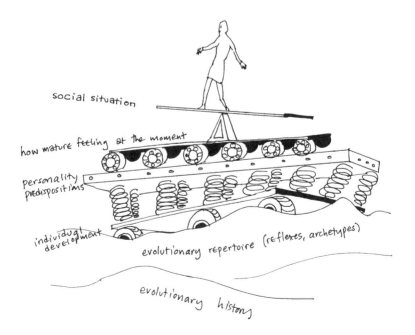

Figure 2.9

3

First stop Babel: advice before embarking

Tribal behaviour likely to be encountered during the excursions, and how it throws light on the nature of consciousness

Let me clarify why I am talking about the Tower of Babel (with the story of the expulsion from the Garden of Eden by way of an introduction to the theme). Since I am basing the arguments in this book on natural rather than supernatural understanding, how can 'religion' or 'mythology' have a place in informing us about the human brain? Because, as said earlier, these stories are products of the human brain, and are as valid as any other accounts which brain scientists put under the general heading 'self-report' data. Moreover, they are 'reports' which have become established in folklore and stories and entered our consciousness; they don't occupy a place 'somewhere else'. Like all memory and archives, they aren't 'past' except in the imagination, but right now, as far as consciousness is concerned.

Myths, like narrative and poetry, may not tell us with precision what brain chemistry or structure is like, but they do demonstrate ways in which it is possible to think (Clocksin 1995). The patient of a psychologist, psychotherapist or psychiatrist also describes ways of thinking, feeling and being – not necessarily immediately helpful to himself, yet important information. Some accounts and tales become repeated, replicated, and mythic and endure over time, and it is reasonable to assume that they began as yarns spun for a purpose (to amuse, inform, warn, or establish the role and esteem of the teller) and some became established because they had some kind of function like 'don't go near the water', or 'don't talk to strange men' which not only – sometimes – proved useful, but also became part of the contents of human consciousness. For good or ill, they were part of a number of narratives that gave the human race ideas of how to be. The process still goes on: the narratives (some true, most transient, much fictional) relating to science, to arts, to academia generally, and to other cultural phenomena such as drama (television, radio, film, theatre), writing (newspapers, magazines, books) and so on complementing what is in the mind so far with the imagery of roles and circumstances and accounts of myriad different ways of being, aspiring and responding. Words, again: as the distinguished quantum physicist Neils Bohr said, faced with the challenge of describing the indescribable, 'we are suspended in language' (Pais 1991). The metaphysical philosopher Martin Heidegger wrote that 'words and language aren't wrappings in which things are packaged for the commerce of those who write and speak. It is in words and language that things first come into being and are.' (Heidegger 1959).

Examples from a helpful ancestor 1: Eden

First, the Garden of Eden, where the serpent persuaded Eve to eat fruit from the Tree of Knowledge, whereupon the bottom fell out of an idyllic world. Lidley, who wrote the 18th C libretto (based on Milton's *Paradise Lost*) of Haydn's otherwise joyful and celebratory oratorio *The Creation*, felt constrained, so it seemed to me, to emphasise a point:

> *O happy pair!*
> *And happy still if not misled by false conceit.*
> *Ye strive for more than granted is;*
> *And more desire to know than know ye should.*

These admonitory words to Adam and Eve are true to the Bible tale about the perils of eating from the Tree of Knowledge. It could hardly be a clearer warning: don't try to know too much. Many contemporary professions, notably in politics and the civil services, adhere firmly to such principles in their dealings with the public. Some nooks and corners of academia, as we have seen, take much the same approach about forbidden knowledge – taboo, with its opposite, the sacred cow.

In *The Prayer of Miriam Cohen*, Rudyard Kipling (1922) gave much the same cautionary advice, though with the characteristic humanity and fine poetry to which he could often rise; he also brought the subject matter somewhat up to date, psychologically speaking.

> *A veil twixt us and thee, good Lord*
> *A veil twixt us and thee*

Lest we should hear too clear, too clear
And unto madness see.

Knowledge, and Knowledge of God, are somehow conflated in these two examples of warnings common in folklore ('you can know too much, you know'), and as you will see as we orbit towards Chapters 9 and 11 this dual-purpose intellectual and spiritual counsel, part admonitory and part helpful, does have a role when we build up our model of consciousness: of how and what we may be and think.

Projecting somewhat, or perhaps regressing, I can imagine some readers becoming impatient with poetic sources and mythology and wanting to get back to the firmer territory, supposedly, of brain structure and function. But if I may invite them to pause and reflect about themselves for a moment, what constitutes your subjective sense of consciousness? Neurochemistry, or buzzing ancestral (and more recent) voices?

Stories, poems, folklore, tales, academic theories and mythology – in which, as Bohr said, we are suspended no less, I think, than our physiological need to be similarly suspended in the right kind of fluid; all these narratives nurture and feed our developing consciousness historically, culturally and individually. They include, naturally, stuff for amusement as well as useful advice, rubbish and communicated craziness. Their evolutionary and cultural function has been to steer what was thought to be a normative course at the time, affirming the group's or tribe's shared common sense and consciousness. The culture developed shamans, priests, leaders, soothsayers, oracles, teachers and no doubt assorted itinerants and drifters all with their roles in this, and the object was partly social control and partly related warnings about what was deemed at the time sensible and sane – for early humans in particular, who had to be careful, an evolutionary imperative. We receive the same today, in newspapers and the 'media' generally, from whoever at any given time form the intellectual elite, in the form of political positions and social and health and safety advice, increasingly backed by law, and in the tales parents tell their children.

Examples from a helpful ancestor 2: Babel

But does it listen, the human race? It does not, and as always seeks to find out for itself: to 'grasp beyond its reach' (Robert Browning [1855] in *Andrea del Sarto*) '– or what's a heaven for?'. Driven by curiosity, increasingly busy, the human race started specialising, initially into hunters and gatherers, child-minders, potters, soldiers and so on, and then into different kinds of story-tellers, priests, shamans and leaders, and, as we will see later, different varieties of eccentric too. Briefly, a reminder of the Babel tale: as the human race journeyed from the East – for which there is DNA (deoxyribonucleic acid) evidence – speaking one language, they paused to build a city with a tower intended to reach to Heaven. God, the story tells us, perceived over-weaning ambition in them and put a spanner in the works by rendering them unable to understand each other.

Ideas, even good ones, may or may not endure or translate into actions. Here the innovative individual faces a rather testing double hurdle from those charged with the task of conserving the culture. The first challenge is that the creative person's ideas may be regarded as woolly, vague, impractical, narrowly ideological and, in general, best either ignored or scoffed at as daft, if not mad, like building the Tower of Babel. At this stage they may simply be dismissed as cranky, or at the other extreme may occasionally attract homicide. But if they look alarmingly like being put into practice, which means political in the broadest sense (i.e. a policy which might catch on), a second challenge is triggered, and the perpetrator/innovator is guided towards one of the three great institutions of culture for the safe disposal of thinkers and innovators as identified by Leach (1976): if not the scaffold, then prisons, mental hospitals or academia, whichever suits.

Now, I have presented this in rather stark though in socio-culturally realistic terms. But human cultures, like the animal kingdom as a whole, are evolved to sense trouble early and deter or deflect it. Thus the religious fundamentalist who applied for an appointment in a scientific department, or my archetypal evolutionary psychologist in an archetypal social science department, would probably not be arrested or sent to a mental hospital; all that would be needed would be a raised eyebrow and a finger discreetly directed at the appropriate part of his or her application, and probably the politest of letters indicating the mismatch between the applicant's qualifications and 'the kind of candidate we are seeking'. Every member of an appointments committee will know as surely as an animal sniffing the air when someone approaching to join the group 'won't be quite right'. The same applies to the agreed curricula, the reading matter selected for the libraries, and so on. For the purposes of discussing how minds work, we do not need to debate whether or not all this is 'good' or 'bad' (*see* again Kleinian theory, p. 12); it is simply how human beings and the institutions we build operate; it is how we are; it is what we do. It is deeply rooted in the type of psychology, group behaviour and neural functioning which provides an early warning system against the thinking, relationships or artefacts which will prove too disturbing for the comfort and balance of the group or institution. The reptile senses the environment, the animal sniffs the air, the higher primate watches for verbal and non-verbal communication: for accents, phraseology, haircut or dress, and one has 'placed' the other, to his or her satisfaction, within a provisional category in a few seconds and within the definitive category only a little later; mad, bad, dangerous to know, or 'not quite one of us'; 'not someone to go into the jungle with'. Such feelings shape cultures.

We cannot tolerate the discordant voices of a Babel, not if we are to get the job done, hence the Babel myth, which, deconstructed, means simply the view that everyone should sing from the same hymn sheet. If we fail to do this, in our Institutions of Psychology, or Psychiatry, or Neuroscience, or Education, or Social Philosophy, or Poetry, or Art, or whatever, the fear is that the Institution itself will deconstruct. This is why the Cautionary Tale has stood the test of time and has been retold and reprinted millions of times; and attributed to God's word (or rationality, or science, or statistics, or convention, or political correctitude) which is handy for leaders and persuaders of every kind.

This is also why, as already said, many a senior academic, indeed of international distinction, in any one of the subjects relevant to human consciousness may know less than an undergraduate or well-read sixth former in another of the core subjects. This is understandable enough; the problem is when he or she *may not want* to know about it, or be contemptuous of the subject.

Searle (1997) reports that in a heated correspondence following a series of articles he wrote about consciousness for the *New York Review of Books* (1995–1997) 'the intensity of feeling bordered on the religious and the political, with more passion from adherents of computational theory than from adherents of traditional religious doctrines of the soul. Some computationalists invest an almost religious intensity into their faith that our deepest problems about the mind will have a computational solution'. Searle suggests that the computer is the latest way of explaining ourselves in accordance with a scientific world view and a new way of understanding ourselves and the possibility of achieving the final technological mastery over human nature. No wonder dissent is upsetting. This, in order to ensure that all hell will not break loose.

Conclusions 1: from Babel

And so we have gone our different ways, speaking languages so different that they attract different kinds of brains (e.g. those which can't cope readily with metaphors on the one hand or mathematics on the other, and cannot comprehend those who can) and the result is that we cannot easily handle communication about the nature of consciousness. This is not (or not entirely) due to human bloody-mindedness and territorial tendencies, but to Consciousness instinctively preserving its integrity by not being too easy to fathom. I'm not sure whether to put it this way is inappropriately anthropomorphic or not. Perhaps anthropomorphism is fitting here? But the point is, I suggest, that this is the way Consciousness works.

I do not intend to criticise academic diversity and dissent, not least because these reflect rather nicely the diversity plus environmental challenge which has got us all the way from insensate chemistry to consciousness. The problem for human and cultural development is not dissenting points of view, but failure even to attempt to understand other views, to discredit them, and to rule them out of the type of academic debate regarded as correct in particular institutions. Now, this is absolutely understandable in intellectual, organisational, institutional and political terms, all highly emotive, competitive areas, but does rather gum up the works if the task is to try to comprehend the nature of consciousness. The specialists and super-specialists need to carry on making their valuable contributions, but there should be another kind of dialogue too, something akin to translation across specialist languages and concepts, and which is seen as strengthening, not weakening, the task of exploring complex ideas. The answer lies in the quality of education, at every level. Some kind of consultative discussion is needed, acknowledging how these cognitive, emotional and institutional barriers can impede education, but such a dialogue requires mutually consenting adults (Steinberg 2005).

Conclusions 2: the uses of ambiguity

i   Consciousness – like art, drama, religion, sex and other forms of man-made magic and high-wire acts – gains by being surrounded by an aura of mystery. This is a deception of sorts, but neither unethical nor impractical because (a) the 'deception' is part of the production, (b) performer and audience agree to collude in the 'deception', and (c) the word 'deception' deserves inverted commas because, as deconstructionist philosophers assert (or even if they didn't), the nature of supposed reality is not that solid: much *is* provisional, subjective and distorted.

ii The need for illusion 'in the theatre', so to speak, does no more than reflect the neuropsychological reality within. You could go through a book letter by letter, but you wouldn't be reading it; you couldn't appreciate a painting by looking only at each particle of pigment through a microscope. This relates to the *gestalt* perspective in psychology ('gestalt' meaning, among other things, form or shape where the whole perception is more than a collection of its constituent parts).

iii Making connections can feel risky. To take two of the familiar extremes, why should the objective and the subjective be regarded as poles apart? Why should religious belief be beyond the pale of normal psychology, as if occupying an inadmissible zone of intellectual thinking? So-called objective, rational scientists and other academics – characteristically thus self-styled – can show, when pressed, remarkable degrees of anxiety and anger if their sense of control over ideas or theory is challenged, even mildly or tangentially. They can be as emotionally driven as any artist, or more so.

Yet we have to be practical too, and in the end, when defining the limits of sanity, of reasonableness, of common sense; even – especially – where we *enlarge* common sense, as the new physics is doing with the cosmos, there is this feeling that we must keep a tighter grip on the subject's boundaries.

In summary: there are conceptual, intellectual, emotional, academic, institutional and traditional reasons why telling a seamless story about consciousness seems next to impossible, and also problems built into the very psycho-physiological and cultural processes by which consciousness is generated. The message in the story of Babel has got us so far, technologically speaking, but for some broad-ranging subjects like the study of consciousness we will have to find the language and the education for connecting what Babel continues to instruct us is unconnectable. But this will take a new revolution in education, and despite all the political rhetoric about 'diversity', 'multi-disciplinary', 'multi-culturalism', 'holism' and so on – which divide as much as they unite – this is at present nowhere in sight.

The story so far

Consciousness is rooted in an inner imagery which relates to past experience, past as well as current perceptions from within and without, and which, to anticipate a later step, becomes self-generating. It is a gradually emergent biological phenomenon which begins with the responsiveness of the organism to its outside world, and as the organism learns, that which began as a primitive responsiveness is gradually and systematically elaborated into the organism's experience of and capacity for impacting on that world. The evolutionary component involves (a) the individual organism's inheritance of previous generations' predispositions, (b) variation in these predispositions and (c) the reality that some of them are more favourable to survival and reproduction than others. It is assumed that emergent consciousness is as susceptible to such evolutionary processes as any other of the organism's variables, and while adaptation begins with physical survival, the latter, up the evolutionary scale, increasingly depends on developing social skills and achieving whatever is the prevailing consensus about sanity in an increasingly complex existence. Complex, because once we reach the environments humans elaborate around themselves, kinds of relationships, kinds of ideas, kinds of feelings, kinds of attitudes, kinds of behaviour and kinds of information and communication systems – memories, fantasies, meanings and narratives – all begin to influence the life and capabilities of individuals. The neural structure needed to develop these is adaptive and inherited by the species and becomes the point where what are complex *predispositions* in the genes and brain connect with *actualities* in the culture.

Hence the mind/cultural reciprocity proceeds, and shapes consciousness as surely as do our material brains.

4

The genie in the genes: how chemicals could become conscious

How evolution and time led to a most extraordinary development

An apparently inauspicious beginning

First, a little about that famous birthplace of ours, where the human race still finds itself only too often: in the soup. Given amino acids detected in the primeval ooze, a dispassionate observer could be forgiven for supposing that the idea that these damp chemicals might one day evolve systems that enabled its descendants to speak, to claim a Self, and indeed to become biologists, would go beyond the wildest excesses of science fiction. You certainly wouldn't gamble on the possibility. But consider that well-worn, half-serious thought-experiment, that if you gave a monkey writing equipment and an infinity of time to make marks it would eventually write the plays of Shakespeare. Well, we, or at least one of us, did, and the sonnets too. Nor did it need infinity, but only a few million years from the first hominids to the great dramatist. However, even given the power of Darwinian theory many feel that there has not been enough time for us to develop from chemicals. I think this is partly due to a profound and subjective misapprehension about time itself.

Ideas being put forward about models rooted in mathematics by which adaptive evolution could be speeded up, for example by Kirschner and Gerhart's review (2005), represent an important field of enquiry; but I also think we underestimate the difficulty of conceptualising the unimaginable lengths of time involved when we speak of *three thousand million* years of the evolution of life on earth. I doubt whether the human mind can realistically comprehend a million years, let alone three thousand million. Also, at least as far as consciousness is concerned, I think we underestimate how much spadework has been done for us over that kind of period by our very lowly ancestors; even single-celled ones. As we shall see, even the most sophisticated sounding Freudian theory – for many people accompanied by the image of educated middle-class ladies in furs visiting Freud's Vienna consulting room – is not so very far (give or take a few thousand million years) from the existence of single-celled organisms, provided one is prepared to accept a conceptual model of layer upon layer of gradual physical development, and dawning awareness of this development, steadily building up to a kind of palimpsest of what and how we are today.

This is what Sigmund Freud said:

> the whole psychic organism corresponds exactly to the body which, though individually varied, is in all essential features the specifically human body which all men have. In its development and structure, it still preserves elements that connect it with the invertebrates and ultimately with the protozoa. Theoretically it should be possible to 'peel' the collective unconscious, layer by layer, until we come to the psychology of the worm, and even of the amoeba. (Freud 1927)

That is the model for this book, and I think it requires a brief overview before going into it in more detail.

Chemistry to consciousness in ten steps; or making a biochemist from biochemicals

1   Organic chemicals with self-replicating properties formed from inorganic chemicals.
2   Survival of some depended on them being more or less in particular places (e.g. forming on rocks) and in other ways developing boundaries within which their self-replication worked. The cell membrane was the highest form of this ability to contain an environment that would prove advantageous, and both excluded yet kept at hand, for example for nutrition, external supplies. (An early and entirely organic version of ambivalence towards the external world?) This is already not so very unlike survival in the wild in a primitive tent or in a space or diving suit, yet we still have up to a three thousand million year ancestry in which to develop and fine-tune our skills and consciousness.
3   All subsequent evolutionary and creative development is based on the same basic template as that of our amoeba-like ancestor, and this is very broadly consistent with the repetition at higher

and higher levels of natural patterns as described by Mandelbrot (1977) (*see* p. 63). To take in through a permeable but nonetheless protective barrier life sustaining and reproduction-sustaining materials, and reject those that threaten these things, sets a pattern for what follows in the next three thousand million years (*see* p. 103).

4   Next came the development of the most primitive nervous systems, necessary to maintain connections between parts as single-celled animals became more elaborate; though it has been recently suggested that there might have been primitive, microtubular nervous function initiating adaptation and learning even at the protozoan stage (Penrose 2004; *see* p. 185).

All organisms could be placed on a spectrum beginning with being simply responsive to the outside world and then becoming in some way sensate in a rudimentary way, much as a spider in a web (or an intruder alarm system) is sensate and responsive, and with higher animals still this led to something we regard as 'awareness', a phenomenon on the fringe of human consciousness. It would require something like true memory (not just learning) to make this leap from mere inner representation of the outside world, and I doubt whether a spider 'knows', still less 'remembers', that there is a web or a caught fly out there, or a bee 'knows' or 'remembers' that there is a hive across the field. But perhaps a cat, a horse or a dog – for all that we tend to anthropomorphise them – may have a kind of transient but repetitive inner representation that, for example, 'over there' food and warmth is to be had. Do animals that seem to have innate potential for adapting to domestication represent early forms of cultural evolution? Meanwhile, if we track forward from insects and anthropoids, and back from humanity, we find reptiles, even three hundred million years ago (*see* p. 71), which had it in their repertoire, albeit unconsciously, to nurture their young with attention, skill and self-sacrifice. The seeds of what would become 'attachment' (*see* Chapter 5) were in animals even then.

5   Next, three mutually-reinforcing phenomena developed together, as creatures and their nervous systems became more complex; and I suggest we are already within striking distance of higher primates, proto-humanity and man. These were (a) retained imagery – not necessarily only visual, (b) memory, and (c) feelings attached to both.

6   We may suppose that animals have the raw building blocks of feelings, not just pain and fear but something which if we experienced it we would call pleasure, triumph or a sense of domination: the kinds of raw, inchoate materials for proto-emotion (but not yet felt in the human sense) of what it is to chase or be chased, catch or be caught, mate or be mated, eat or be eaten. It is as if such dramas were happening, again in the terms of awareness, in silence, with the lights switched off and no anticipation or memory involved. This was yet to develop.

7   The next big step is the emergence of creatures who survived but who couldn't run all that fast, fly, or camouflage themselves, and whose children are born years from being able to fend for themselves: us. Our growing brains made it necessary for us to be delivered prematurely, in a relatively infantile state, and further survival happened (to those of our ancestors who survived – it was not preordained, remember) because some of us were able to come to some mutually collaborative social arrangement with others: adults with adults, parents with offspring.

The need was still as it was with the single-celled animal: air, water, food, warmth, shelter. Such factors enabled life or caused death; and those who could anticipate a little way ahead, guess or read others' intentions, practise deception and scheme, were at an advantage which they needed, not having huge claws, teeth, wings, poisons and other protective gear. The new brain development helped the new micro-culture; and vice versa. Now, some of this new inner imagery came from within – for example that it perhaps 'didn't feel nice' to be eaten, or kill, or have sex forced on you. But what of the more complex, pro-social imagery from *without*? How could all *that* get into the mind? Given creatures that survive by cooperation and nurturing of children, we will see that attachment theory and the psychology of relationships provide a conceptual model and a route from the developing social circumstances into the psyche.

Thus, there are two crucial cycles: an internal cycle between fleeting experience and memory, turning transient raw emotion into something experienced as feelings and at times recalled as significant; and an external cycle, again 'felt', about what happens in the outside world. This represents the first turning of the carousel to which I referred earlier: that the emerging, primitive mind begins to make something of the world outside (and make things *in* that world, like shelters, plans, relationships) and the world within; this is the beginning of culture, and it begins to feed and develop the mind.

8   Once this starts there is no obvious end to how elaborate it can become, because we are now beyond mere survival and primitive manipulation and deception of others; imagery now becomes imagination and 'what if?' becomes possible – anticipation, fantasy, speculation about alternatives, a whole unstoppable chain reaction of creativity and innovation. Also recollections, with feelings like joy, regret and guilt, become possibilities too, and are powerfully inhibiting or motivational, as our proto-human ancestors become human. In fact these things, incorporating rudimentary reflection, empathy and conscience, *make* us human.

9   Three key phenomena reinforce this kind of emotional development.

i   First, *projection*. This psychoanalytic idea, of the attribution to others and other situations of feelings within oneself, represents another layering on top of what the nervous system can do and of what the locomotor system can do. Referring again to the scene in Kubrick's film *2001* in which the ape, triumphantly discovering a bone as a weapon, flings it into the sky, and the spinning bone is turned cinematographically into a turning space station, this represents what the nervous system can do, what muscles and bones can do, and what the projecting, metaphorical imagination of the film's director can do. Three levels: locomotor, neural, imaginative. We project, literally and metaphorically, ideas, words and things as grappling irons to engage with the world, to see if 'it' (our effort and the world) works. Language might have begun that way – 'throw out' a grunt (for assistance, or for attracting attention to something), to see if anyone out there recognises something by the noise and responds in some way. To the extent that it works, it becomes an emotional, linguistic and cognitive tool in the inside world as well as a piece of language (a small scrap of culture) in the outside world, initiating a mirroring in the other individual, who also learns something linguistic, emotional and cognitive. Bit by bit, such things haul us forward.

ii   The second is *empathy* – not, I suggest, necessarily benign in its basic psychological machinery; one can see in the reading of other people's supposed states of mind (i.e. the throwing out of what A thinks and feels into what A thinks B might think and feel) the seeds and opportunities for manipulation, *Schadenfreude* and sadism too. The accumulation of theories about other people and the outside world – often with not entirely reliable or consistent feedback – generates theories about relationships, which can include trust on the one hand and paranoia on the other. Paranoia is important, and is in its way both potentially creative and potentially damaging: it is essentially about conclusions made by an animal determined to make sense of the world, whatever gaps there are in knowledge, but built upon evidence that may be inadequate. This happens in the best regulated circles.

iii The third phenomenon is the most controversial, the Jungian notion of the *archetype*. Dismissed as said as mystical nonsense and more or less ignored in mainstream science, psychology and psychiatry, yet increasingly consistent with findings in much recent neuroscience and genetic ideas about language, what the archetype represents is argued in Chapter 7. We shall see that archetypal theory can explain how psychosocial developments can be hard-wired into the genes and the brain.

10 What I have proposed here is a route 'up' from lower animals to articulate human beings who can describe their inner fantasies and feelings, and indeed their sense of self. Dennett, comparing mere sentience with human consciousness, noted the two routes, one prospective (ascending sentience), and the other working back from our own 'richly detailed and richly appreciated experience' (Dennett 1991) and he could see no way they could connect – 'like two ships that pass in the night'. This is because of one of the very many regrettable conceptual and linguistic disconnections which have plagued understanding since Babel. Psychodynamic theories of the unconscious provide metaphors for connecting animal functioning with the operations of the unconscious mind, and throw lines (narrative lines as well as metaphorical ropes) from one of Dennett's ships to the other. Freud was primarily a biologist (Sulloway 1979), aware of the ingesting, excreting, reproducing, pain-avoiding, comfort-seeking animal in man. Jung (1954) took things further into the kind of lives, myths and culture the human race began to build about itself, like a pro-cultural nest. The attempts by both (like Neils Bohr (Bohr 1963; Pais 1991)) to render complex, pre-verbal abstractions into language have been ill-served by the less imaginative and open minded, who reject metaphor and symbolism that they can't comprehend

while they would not have the presumption to reject equally baffling mathematical concepts.

There are, then, aspects of theories of unconscious functioning which will serve as links between developing animal sentience and the contemporary human mind, and in Chapter 9 I will propose a tentative model, mediated by findings in neuroscience, as to how this connection can account for a sense of self and the emergence of the elusive 'I'; bearing in mind that none of the above yet accounts for this 'I', since we have not yet established a system for there being in one place 'Io' (p. 31): that is, both inner imagery, however elaborate, and its observer.

5

A fateful attachment

Family life: from necessities to niceties

Strange situations

I have been arguing that a neural account of the conscious mind provides an essential but insufficient explanation of the 'I', and that to make progress in completing the picture we must incorporate experiences from without (the material world) and from within. But how does such experience get into the nerve networks? I have drawn attention to our amoeba-like ancestors, taking in, excreting and making something of themselves, albeit in the unconscious dark. We do the same, literally and metaphorically, as we develop consciousness, and crucial to this is the development of inner imagery.

Where do images come from? And how to they 'get in'? Not by simple perception and memory alone, because the imagery I am talking about is heavily affect-laden and suffused with meaning, so must gain something from the nascent psyche. This happens primarily through relationships which at this level of sophistication are unique to the human world; our survival has depended on imagery in the head that helps us find our way around in the three worlds: an emerging inner world, the material outer world, and the world of relationships, and for this John Bowlby's attachment theory provides a model that straddles evolutionary biology, psychology, philosophy and social science (Bowlby 1969, 1973, 1979; Holmes 1993; Knox 2003), although in this account I have amplified the prominence he gave to the development of inner imagery. Through relationships the emergent, self-conscious individual-to-be must also develop some sense of being, time and place.

Discussing the evolution of the mind requires us to think in three phases. First, and 'hard-wired' within us, as something adaptive which was learned by our ancestors and with which we are born. We should not take for granted our first perceptions, recognition and response to other creatures; it requires a mechanism, and some of it is innate. Second, this continues to develop from childhood onwards, and has been studied through primate and human group observations and in experimentally contrived 'strange' (i.e. new, unfamiliar) situations. Third – and this steps beyond Bowlby's initial notion of attachment theory – how it applies during the whole of the rest of our lives, in big events and small. I have already referred to these stages, which you might conceive of as three sliding scales, on page 44. In order to understand the emotive potential of imagery, however, it is necessary to say a brief word about the psychodynamic notion of regression – a slipping back on our sliding scale. In a sentence: a mature, competent person under sufficient stress can slip back to a most immature way of feeling and responding. As mentioned earlier, anyone looking after the public know this – waiters and waitresses, police officers, and airline staff coping with a clientele regularly balanced on the cusp of high hopes and anxiety in a strange situation if ever there was one (*see* Figure 5.1). As mentioned elsewhere, how the individual reacts isn't tied to his or her chronological age or apparent maturity, because shifting back and forth around this point is part of the dynamic of fluctuating self-management in fluctuating situations.

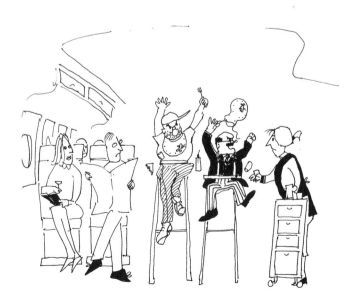

Figure 5.1

The importance of making connections

'Only connect the prose and the passion', wrote E M Forster in *Howard's End* (1910), 'and both will be exalted'. With Burnshaw (1982) I would like to try to connect biological necessity with metaphor and emotion; and attachment theory, linking as it does evolution with imagery and relationships, provides a possibly viable point of contact. Just as the exigencies of single-celled life make, literally, the first moves (towards, away from) and provide hypothetical foundations for attraction, repulsion, the dynamics of attachment make feasible the generation on both sides of imagery and feelings with which we are familiar (love, hate, dependence, independence, gratitude, resentment) and the need to put them into words. Given time and the repetition of simple patterns of behaviour to ever greater levels of complexity, basic needs (a gnawed bone) can become the superficially sophisticated dinner party.

Or the advantages of meiosis metamorphose into the incest taboo. It may appear fanciful to relate sexual reproduction (meiosis) at the cellular level to species behaviour. But it was meiosis that enabled the mixing of genes and diversity that could not happen in asexual reproduction (i.e. identical cloning) and diversity being the first essential step in evolution it is conceivable that sexual reproduction at the single cell level acts in reciprocity with sexual reproduction at the behavioural level, which, if you add to this the complex, cultural rites, rituals and sophistication associated with sex, makes the idea of our 'learning' from the protozoan not all that far fetched. Thus the possible remote roots of the widespread inhibitions, personal as well as cultural, on sexual relationships between close relatives. Again, we should not read that the wrong way round: the taboo didn't 'prevent' incest; it is more likely that incestuous relationships didn't do well, in terms of descendants, and those with a taboo which might have been in the minority and regarded as anomalous ended up with the most descendants.

I think we shouldn't leave out senses of time and place when considering connectedness. We establish useful connections and disconnections when we climb a tree to escape a predator, climb up a parent for love or protection, make a primitive boat (and persuade others to join us) to see if there is food on the other side of the river, and when we 'pursue' a career or something else important in life. It is good that we have the notion of 'being somewhere else sometime' within us.

Further, one of the most persisting themes in understanding the roots of creativity and innovation has been the juxtaposition of ideas or things that had previously been separated, from tool-making and engineering to all the arts

Culturally and academically, attempts to 'connect up' paradoxically require a sense of difference (indeed valuing difference) before connections are made to produce (as in meiosis) something different from both original sources. Humanity has benefited vastly from focused, convergent, categorising, objective, specialist thinkers and workers, even though going too far in that direction can make the useful connections perceived by divergent, intuitive, fuzzy, impressionistic thinkers and workers difficult to appreciate. If the message of Babel was 'specialise' rather than have your head in the clouds, that has certainly been useful for us; but there is something about the needs and tentative thinking of the times, from science through medicine to ecology and to how cultures work, that makes me feel that after several hundred years of 'contraction' and scientific and technical advance a period of 'expansion' is due. Perhaps there's another myth to support this. The only narrative, or myth, at present, and an influential one, comes back to attachment and collaboration: that artists and scientists inhabit two irreconcilably different cultures.

Does connecting up to enable biological, social and cultural development fit in with Mandelbrot's accounts of the organisation of the physical world in repetitive fractal patterns at very different levels of organisation (Mandelbrot 1977)? It is the way a trickle of water on the sand reproduces a vast estuary, or the pattern is seen in the structure of the veins of a leaf; it is the way the physical world works, and may colour the way we work too.

But back to the basics of attachment theory. Essentially this chapter describes a process by which an immature animal, which is potentially emotionally isolated, establishes connections –relationships – with caring, experienced adults, and this not only makes survival possible, but shows it how to establish relationships with future others, to mate, and to have progeny; and to relate sufficiently well to its offspring for them to survive and reproduce too. I have widened the theme, however, to see in the inner and outward exploration made possible by attachment theory significance also for exploring new ideas and new connections – even if they seem strange. That too takes care, containment and confidence.

What is attachment theory?

John Bowlby was one of the few towering figures in the psychiatry of the second half of the twentieth century, and among the pioneers who sought to integrate psychoanalytic theory, clinical experiences with families and the findings of ethologists – animal behaviourists who tried to explain how and (in evolutionary terms) why certain patterns of animal behaviour developed. The focus of the work of Bowlby and his collaborators became the way the human infant developed behaviourally, emotionally and intellectually as a result of the close bond formed between the child and the mother or other caregiver. This was mutual – the child had an innate predisposition to keep close to a caring adult and the adult a reciprocal predisposition to respond. Flaws in such reciprocity, apart from threatening survival (in both evolutionary terms and in individual development) could also produce depressive states, rooted in a profound sense of abandonment and loss, anxiety and aggressive states, and personality disorders. The notion of 'childhood trauma' causing problems later causes a lot of misunderstanding, for two main reasons. It is not usually a 'sudden trauma' which affects children so much as the persistent failure of care and upbringing. Children are very adaptive and resourceful, but sustained parental neglect or mishandling eventually wears them down. Emotional growth takes sustained work and skill on the part of those caring for them, and this is what attachment theory is about.

Earlier I described the importance of systems and cycles of events, since they explain living systems better than simple linear ('A leads to B') conceptual models. The evidence is that they describe better what actually happens. One sees these actually operating in clinical work (Steinberg 2000, 2005; Tyrer and Steinberg 2005), because while the individual psychodynamic model proposes psychological processes going on as if 'in the head' (*see* Figure 5.2), in therapeutic work with families and groups the processes may be observed before you – in the head and in the room. Take for example a patient who says he feels a 'failure'; and one can imagine, if one isn't careful, a kind of 'failure complex' composed of wrong thinking and mood problems existing in his head like some kind of phantom tumour. In a group, however, particularly in family work, one may see one child, for example, encouraged by one or both parents to be the family extrovert, clown and favourite ('just look at him – come on down from the doctor's filing cabinet, Craig') while his big sister is given the role of serious, perfectionist scholar embodying the family's ambitions – until she develops anorexia nervosa, which 'really' lets everyone down. Thus interpersonal behaviour explains and complements what is 'in the head' (*see* Figure 5.3).

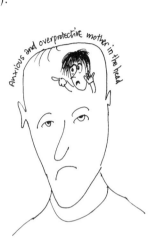

Figure 5.2

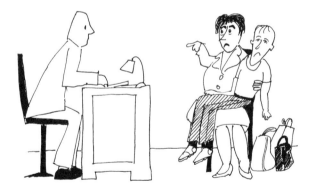

Figure 5.3

Once individuals are in these roles, by now integral to self-identity, it can be difficult to change them, to get a new part in the drama – the boy to take himself more seriously and relate non-competitively to his sister, the anorexic daughter to be herself instead of being a repository of parental ambitions, and (as may well be seen in a clinic) the father to cut down on his workaholism and alcoholism and help his wife with her isolation and sadness. Many family therapists work directly with such mutually entrapping behaviour without speculating on what may be happening in the unconscious mind. Such mutually reinforcing or undermining cycles of behaviour also operate in the opposite way too: encouraging and supporting each other, enhancing self-esteem and dealing appropriately with problems. However, the allotment of roles, and their unthinking acceptance, isn't only a clinical phenomenon. It is how the human race carries on, producing 'leaders', 'failures', 'stars', friends, enemies, all the *dramatis personae* of our existence and our cultures.

In attachment theory we have a descriptive model for what is going on socially between people, and also for what is going on in their heads, in terms of learned and prevailing feelings and attitudes. In order to explain it, we should first consider some of the ideas in psychodynamic theory from which it grew.

Psychoanalytic theory is widely criticised for relying on evidence from Freud's and his followers' introspection and imagination, and reporting what their patients 'introspected' too. Criticised as purely intuitive, speculative and subjective, we should however note the view by the philosopher Henri Ey (Evans 1972) that objectivity about subjective feelings should not be regarded as inadmissible. Evans' paper was turned down by the prominent psychiatric journals of the day, and published instead in the harder-headed and prestigious neurological journal *Brain* (Evans, personal communication). So we will consider attachment theory in the light of its Freudian ancestry.

Freud and some of his followers; in five short steps

1   Sigmund Freud (1856–1939), physician, biologist and neuro-scientist, established a theory he called psychoanalysis. From it developed a number of schools of thought generally known as psychodynamic theory or depth psychology. It concerns the effect on our thinking and behaviour patterns of feelings of which we are ordinarily unaware, and which consequently generate attitudes, imagery and imaginings (fantasies) whose origins aren't ordinarily accessible in our day-to-day awareness. Hence it is a theory of the unconscious. Psychodynamic refers again to circular rather than linear causation: processes act upon each other and in turn modify those actions so that a general outcome can represent

many internally competing influences. However, these are perceived as primarily acting 'within' the mind, not as in the family's overt behaviour described earlier.

It is important for the person new to the field to know that many apparently quite thoughtful and rational people in the psychological and psychiatric fields regard this approach as rubbish, nonsense, pernicious and even crazy. Foucault (1967), Marxist philosopher and no natural ally of psychoanalysis, nevertheless allowed that Freudian theory at least made possible a 'dialogue with unreason', which within the limits of his cautious recommendation is good enough.

2 The *Unconscious* is seen as the repository of material which is influential on the conscious mind but concealed there because the conscious mind finds it inadmissible in terms of unthinkable thoughts and unacceptable feelings. However, they can become conscious, or part-conscious, or near-conscious, or conscious in a distorted kind of way, for example in psychoanalytic exploration, in symbolic form in fantasies and dreams, in their contribution to artistic expression, and in such accidents as slips of the tongue.

What the Unconscious actually 'is' is hard to say; and some behavioural psychologists, irrationally I think, regard the notion of an 'unconscious mind' as an oxymoron. (There is however some superficial validity if a scientist claims that the only data relevant to 'science' is that which is measurable, and that the only psychological phenomenon that you can take a calculator to is behaviour.) On the other hand, remember that the physical functioning of our nerve cells, while presumably relevant here, is also unconscious. Later, I will try to argue that the unconscious mind, far from being a kind of weird dark cellar, often closed off from our conscious minds, is in fact as active, productive, immediate and relevant as, say, the soil is to a farm or garden.

3 How do the unconscious contents of the mind get there? Psychodynamic theory proposes a whole battery of defence mechanisms (e.g. repression, suppression, denial) by which the conscious mind defends itself from awkward, unwelcome or even horrifying material; the kinds of thing we label 'thinking the unthinkable' or 'I couldn't live with myself if I thought that', and so on; indeed crazy, asocial, surreal stuff. But much of it was there anyway, indeed preceded the emergence of the relatively civilised, sociable mind. Freud suggested three components of the mind: the *Id*, or 'it', the raw, basic animal mind, laid down as suggested earlier all

the way from the amoeba to the ape; the *Super-ego*, where what the wild Id wants (food, sex, space) has to come to terms with the constraints of social expectations, learned, painfully, as primates found it was necessary to be diplomatic and to allow for other people. The *Ego* – the 'I' – is a kind of homeostatic compromise between the Id and Super-ego. But central though the Ego is in psychoanalytical thinking, the nature of the self-conscious, essential 'I' has been more the province of existential philosophy and consciousness studies than psychodynamic theory which rather takes the mysterious essence of 'I' for granted.

4   One criticism of psychodynamic theory is that it is about what is supposed to go on inside the head, yet what happens (like acquiring the Super-ego) is in fact related to social and cultural expectations and pressures. In therapy too, and in the rest of real life, the theory jumps the gap between one person and another in the form of what Freud called *transference* when feelings deriving from a past problem become attributed to the other person in a new relationship. This is best known, especially in the romantic literature of the 1930s and 1940s, as the patient 'falling in love with the therapist'. In fact it is the *projection* onto other people of all sorts of redundant and semi-redundant past feelings, in which connection a good working definition of a neurosis is that it is a pattern of feeling and behaviour that once had some usefulness or relevance (e.g. childish behaviour, anxiety about something strange) but which in the mature person and grown-up situation should be redundant. For example, attributing to a work colleague or acquaintance feelings acquired in an earlier, long-past relationship, such as a parent who could not be trusted.

5   As a fifth step I will simply mention the other schools of thought or derivations from the basic Freudian theory (see also Brown 1961; Storr 1989). In particular, I will be drawing on ideas from CG Jung (Progoff 1953; Jacobi 1968; Stevens 1990; Storr 1998), Melanie Klein (Hinshelwood 1994) and Jacques Lacan (Benvenuto and Kennedy 1986; Leader and Groves 1995). The whole field is more complicated and riven with controversy than I have indicated, and as already said much of it or all of it is dismissed out of hand by some. It also has to be said that Freudians, Jungians, Kleinians and Lacanians have their huge differences too, and act far from reasonably and with insight in their dealings with each other. For all this it is a rich, instructive literature and makes a real contribution to understanding the mind; to dismiss it is rather like

saying art has nothing to do with politics – it depends on the art and on the politics. I would like to give the literary critic Harold Bloom the last word at this point. Clearly troubled by the notion of Freud as a scientist, he observed:

he is no more a charlatan than the Socrates of Plato's symposium ... throwing Freud out will not get rid of him, because he is inside us. His mythology of the mind has survived his supposed science, and his metaphors are impossible to evade. (Bloom 2002)

These are the barest bones of the Freudian approach, indeed not all the bones. For further reading I would recommend Freud (1952, 1954, 1959), Wollheim (1971), Sulloway (1979), Stafford-Clark (1983) and Storr (1989).

The relevance of Freudian theory to a model for the conscious mind

The aspects of psychoanalytic theory I want to extract because of their usefulness as connections with a new model for the conscious mind are:

(a) that for the 'unconscious mind' read an animal mind being nudged by adaptive necessity and growing complexity towards pro-social behaviour and the beginnings of culture and inner and outer awareness – particularly the former

(b) that the conscious, civilised, 'sophisticated' mind is constantly capable of slipping back (regression) into primitive attitudes and modes of feeling, operating highly selectively (e.g. denial), projecting feelings onto other people, and deceiving the self

(c) that the 'unconscious mind' is no mere below-stairs appendage of a much more impressive 'consciousness', but is an integral part of the whole. This is relatively unexplored territory in consciousness studies.

(d) that (*vide* Bloom, above) the incorporation in our thinking of Freudian metaphors (if you can swallow them) is one example of an infinity of ways in which the productions of influential minds and brains contribute to the way subsequent minds think, thereby completing the mind development/cultural development cycle: minds make thoughts which make language and culture, and these shape developing minds.

The unconscious mind and its biology

But – continuing from point (d) – this is not a simple process. Blackmore's and Dawkins' idea of 'memes' (Dawkins 1976; Blackmore 2002) – a whole teeming memosphere, if I may call it that – of ideas and artefacts may not, I think, be truly analogous to natural selection in the way they suggest; but it does constitute a nice metaphor for a never-ending torrent of other people's replicated ideas pouring into the culture and helping establish our minds from countless sources – everything, round the clock, from ordinary conversation to the 'media', and occupying every conceivable kaleidoscopic modality – words, symbolism, music, habits, fashion, information and imagery of every kind. They are copied by imitation and teaching and selected (or not) by our memory, and as huge, intrapsychic complexes. Blackmore (1999, 2002) suggests they form an illusion of the self. I don't think they do, alone, but – to use Boorstin's (2001) analogy of imaginative, creative people having 'enlarged, embellished, fantasized and filigreed our experience' – I think they build upon the latticework of the self which emerges from the unconscious and is then drawn out by our relationships.

This cultural and subcultural contribution to the way minds function represents one aspect of a complex process by which the external world, both 'made' and natural, 'gets in'. But for the moment I want to consider how its complementary half, the unconscious, arises in the mind. In putting it this way I am going to suggest that the animal life I will be referring to is, in the human sense, mindless. It is sensate, responsible, 'aware' in the way that electronic detection equipment may be said, anthropomorphically, to be sensing something in the environment and reacting to it; but in terms of anything approaching consciousness all this takes place in the dark, in a kind of existential vacuum.

The model I am going to propose for the proto-mind (the building bricks of that which will in humans become mind) is of powerful and imperative physiological events and activities (like catching live prey and consuming it – or like being caught and eaten) that provide phenomena which millions, or thousands of millions, of years later became experienced by a conscious mind. In other words: what would it feel like to be an amoeba, moving through environments which represent gradients of wetness and dryness, nutrition and toxicity, coldness and warmth? Ingesting and excreting as it goes? Can you imagine?

On the narrow gap I am postulating between the amoeba and our sophisticated selves, I wonder if any reader has ever been drunk or otherwise intoxicated, for example by illness or medication? The hypothetical reader could be the biochemist referred to earlier (evolved from organic chemicals) or a philosopher or an accomplished pianist and an international expert on, say, chess or a small area of Chinese pottery. But it doesn't take very much in the way of an alteration in brain chemistry or temperature (the parameters are quite narrow) for the most finely honed mind to regress to a state of lying very still under the blankets, consciousness closed down to total preoccupation with trying or hoping to feel better and anxious not to feel worse, and nothing else (yesterday, tomorrow, others, all the memes) being of interest at all. In such states even a sense of time may be distorted, the person concerned being not only disorientated but experiencing his or her limited world in fleeting, transient half-grasped scenes. Infantile, dependent behaviour is common here too. Although, in most such states, a few days pass and our near-vegetative, amoebic creature is sitting up and finishing *The Times'* crossword.

All the way up the evolutionary scale, our 'earlier' brains are still within us, there to be anatomically delineated. The reptilian brain (primarily the basal ganglia) evolved three hundred million years ago, and was then added to by the paleo-mammalian brain (primarily the limbic system with its endocrine connections) and then the neo-mammalian brain, the neo-cortex, which operates less instinctively and is more concerned with cognition. These components make up what MacLean (1985) called the triune brain, 'each with its own phylogenetic (evolutionary) history and each with its own special sense of time and space and its own motor functions' (MacLean 1985; Stevens and Price 1996).

I would like to select from this intriguing material two examples, one an aspect of reptilian functioning and the other an aspect of avian functioning which I will identify as 'mindless', yet which laid the foundations, hundreds of millions of years ago, for what far more recently became incorporated in the attachment behaviour of primates – and ourselves.

Early reptiles were able to show what we would (anthropomorphically again) identify as nurturing behaviour. For example Dimetrodon, which lived three hundred million years ago, would not only put herself at risk by guarding her eggs, eating little and remaining vulnerably in one place, but is thought to have modified the temperature of her eggs by painstakingly adjusting the amount of cover they had. This creature also had meat-shearing teeth like our own and a large spinal 'sail' for modifying body temperature. She was not our ancestor, evolutionary ancestry being multi-branched. But mid-way, one might say, between the amoeba and ourselves, the branching evolutionary stream carried to us the seeds of mammalian and then primate nurturing behaviour: all of it quite unconscious.

The other example is more up to date. Today's newspapers (Christmas 2005) contain accounts of Kyala and Oscar, two blackfoot penguins in an Isle of Wight zoo, pining for a missing infant, Toga. The mother penguin is eating only enough to survive, and with her mate explores every nest-box many times a day in the hope of finding the baby. Much as I am a lover of animals, I do not believe that these penguins are experiencing what we would experience if dressed up in penguin-suits and looking for a lost child. Again, sadly, I fear it all takes place in relative emotional darkness. I am not saying these birds feel nothing; there is no doubt some kind of raw, moment-by-moment experience, just as in other circumstances an animal shows rage or fear. But it is not accompanied by memories, fantasies, fearful or hopeful anticipations, mixed feelings and self-reference ('I'll never forgive myself for taking my eye off him for that moment', etc.). But this is not to devalue these proto-emotional states: they make us what we are; are in us now, as part of our unconscious repertoire, but elaborately built upon with memory, imagery, words, metaphors and meaning.

Arousal: mediating perception, stimulus and emotion

I will briefly enlarge on arousal, having suggested the idea as something in animals that could be 'not-quite-feeling'. In a classic experiment by Schachter and Singer (1962) volunteers were given adrenalin or a placebo and exposed (in what they thought was a waiting area, but was in fact the experiment) to an actor among them who acted playfully or angrily. Essentially, those on adrenalin and exposed to the 'fun' actor became more or less euphoric, and those exposed to the provocateur became angry, while those on a placebo were not markedly affected. This relatively simple experiment suggests a connection between simple arousal and the elicitation of more complex, subtle feelings by the prevailing social situation, and provides a possible connection between unconscious physiological changes and conscious culturally-determined feelings. It may not be much; but it is a possible link in the chain.

Arousal to cognition

Parkes (1969), a collaborator of John Bowlby who has studied grief in humans and its equivalent in animals, has described certain patterns of behaviour in response to significant loss in terms of changes in behaviour due to the 'absence of stimuli on which the original behaviour depended'. This sounds cold, compared with, say, a mother's grief, but again it describes the basics of biological loss: the mother animal has a whole range of experience, behaviour and response stimulated by the presence of the infant; and when the infant is lost a 'hole' appears in this repertoire of experience, behaviour and response. As conscious humans we feel this 'hole' only too well, reflect on it, fantasise about it, try to cope with it in adaptive and maladaptive ways, try to fill the gap in our understanding as well as in our feelings and behaviour, and then 'fix' it with the word 'grief'. Parkes describes the actual *behaviour* of an animal which has lost its young in terms of agitated, searching, restless behaviour, crying out, preoccupation with any conceivable sign or signal of the missing infant; this is extraordinarily like human grief, even to the grieving person's heightened perception of the lost person, thinking again and again that they have glimpsed them in crowds. The literal (and adaptive) 'search for a lost object', in terms of observable behaviour, is the same as the psychoanalytical metaphor for grief, but arrived at independently, and in another scientific era, by intuitive, reflective speculation about clinical cases of grief and depression.

One more experiment possibly connecting our different kinds of brain to different patterns of behaviour: Gregory (1970, 1997, 2005) has described an extraordinary 'hollow mask' experiment based on the illusion in which observers of the concave side of a face mask cannot, despite their best visual efforts, perceive the nose of the mask as indented. It invariably appears to project, because we know that is what noses do. However, when experimental subjects are asked to very quickly touch the tip of the nose without thinking, their fingers go straight to the true (indented) tip, not the illusory one. Gregory attributed this to the difference between how a reflex perception (such as a reptile, or our reptilian brain) would perform, and a perception based on a concept of what a face is supposed to be like. Our brain, emerging into consciousness, abhors a vacuum. Visually, emotionally, cognitively we fill gaps, try to make sense, whatever the amount of information we have to go on. In this sense I think creativity and paranoia (what was that noise? what did he mean by that?) are related, connected by the restless imagination.

Attachment theory

We will therefore be looking at attachment theory from three particular perspectives.

1   First, it represents a crucial evolutionary step which enables helpless human infants to survive by developing social relationships, rather than by more basic animal protection such as camouflage, hiding, fight and flight.
2   Second, I will argue that the socially determined, behavioural imperatives of attachment behaviour – the necessary relatedness of infant to caregivers – acts as a spur to dawning consciousness of the external world and the world within, and modifies simple reflex perceptions into those that are cognitively more elaborate, indeed pro-cultural, and having survival value reappear in descendants just as a simple protective reflex would.
3   Third, that the raw proto-emotional material brought into this affective hothouse is essentially the same as the *unconscious* repertoire of animal arousal and responses described earlier.

Imagine two scenes, about a million years apart, though only two or three thousand miles in terms of space. The earlier scene is somewhere in North Africa, perhaps not far from Baghdad, where some of humanity's early story-tellers placed the Garden of Eden. For the present scene, imagine a park in a city centre. In Scene One a proto-human and her offspring are gathered in a space between trees, cliffs and water. The young are playing; the mother has one infant clamped to her breast, is chewing something, and keeping a watchful eye on the others. One infant wanders towards the trees and is brought sharply back by a mutual glance that flashes between the mother and the child. Another, nearly the same age and hopping about eagerly and intent on following his brother, is knocked over, not too harshly, with a clump from the mother. But one of the daughters, crawling about and fiddling around with some bits of twig and bone a little way off, seems to be playing safely, and whatever passes between her and her mother enables her to carry on with her game; no need to come back is the mutually understood message; but don't go further.

Astonishingly, considering as Dawkins (1998) reminds us of the odds against survival, the remote descendants of this family are now having a picnic in a city park. What is so surprising is the number of the perils negotiated during the intervening million years, and the picnickers owe even the mere feasibility of survival to the development in primates of attachment behaviour. The modern mother is reading a book, but with an eye on the children. The smallest one is kept beside her, and as he can crawl is gently hauled back every so often. The others are playing a little way off. One, interested in some music coming from a clump of bushes, wanders towards the sound and pauses, looking round, to see if her mother will react. The mother doesn't seem to be alarmed, and the child goes a little further, but then spots a dog. It is on a lead, but she isn't too sure about it. The dog is signalling boisterousness – nothing more, nothing less. The dog's owner conveys – without saying anything – something that makes the child's mother appreciate that the dog is OK but ... there is something about the dog's owner's manner and appearance for this mother that urges a little caution. The child looks interested in the dog but holds back. The mother calls to the child, who toddles back to her mother. The mother and the dog's owner exchange a few words. The dog is brought over, picked up, and the child strokes it. Not a lot has happened, but the child is safe, has had a good experience, and furthermore the trajectory of the child's development (through hundreds of such small interactions each day) will influence, eventually, how much the child grows up confident, accident-prone or nervous about dogs or for that matter strangers and adventures. The child may be someone who would dash around a noisy fairground by themselves, or cling to parents. Thousands of alternative scenarios and outcomes could be imagined. With the proto-human family group of a million or so years earlier the mutual interaction was more directly a matter of life and death; now such parental–child mutuality and fine-tuning could influence all manner of emotional and behavioural outcomes. Earlier I referred to the continuing attachment dynamic in adult relationships. In this vignette, something about the stranger has reassured the mother, who has within her a good working balance between trust and caution, and she is able to reassure her child sufficiently for the small social experiment of petting the dog to take place. The attachment dynamic is infectious.

What attachment theory provides is a model for the caretaking adult and the developing infant. It is a dynamically interacting system of capacities and behaviours, which is to say that each modulates the others. The separated components are:

i   that the child's behavioural repertoire includes keeping close enough to an adult who can take care of it ('PSAB', or proximity-seeking attachment behaviour)
ii that the adult's behavioural repertoire includes recognising, and responding to, a younger animal that needs care taken of it ('CT', or caretaking behaviour) (*see* Figure 5.4)
iii the infant's propensity to explore its environment (E) (and *see* Figure 5.5)
iv the infant's ability to construct an internal image of the outside world – one that will work (Io – *see* pp. 31,79).

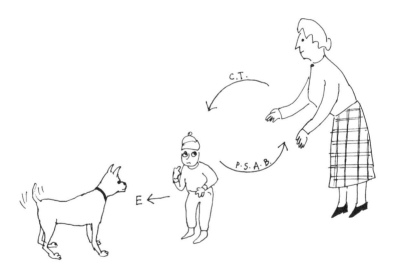

Figure 5.4   Tentative exploration

Like many other things in this book (consciousness, time, survival) the attachment dynamic can be taken too readily for granted. We may say that 'of course' adults look after their young or we wouldn't be here, which is true; however, we consider it obvious because we are

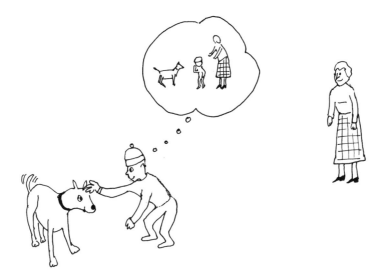

Figure 5.5   Confident exploration

the survivors. The picnic in the park requires gravity too, also taken for granted, but for the purposes of this book we are not yet examining gravity (though *see* pp. 149,183). The nature of life and evolution suggests that there were, down the ages, parents and children who didn't have in their natures the innate, neural fundamentals of what it takes to foster attachment, so they didn't have offspring that survived to reproduce. Those who did, perhaps an odd minority, were the thin straggling line that came, it seems, out of Africa and became our great-great- (to the power of x) grandparents. And yet within the complex, dynamic weave that makes us human, the nurturing dynamic may not survive every social and psychological vicissitude; in particular kinds of socio-cultural deprivation throughout the world, adult attachment breaks down and the breakdown of adult–child attachment follows, and we see neglect, abuse and infanticide emerge only too readily. The attachment dynamic gives us opportunities, not guarantees.

(i) Keeping close to a caretaking adult

If the infant didn't get this right, or (as we are talking about biology too) if something neuropsychological in its behaviour meant that it couldn't get it right, however much help it got, it would have been left to fend for itself in the bush or become hopelessly clinging. Neither would have been likely to lead to survival. On the one hand, it is hard to imagine a proto-human infant standing a chance of finding and providing its own food, warmth, shelter and self-protection in the wild until it was at least seven or eight years old, even if it had been successfully weaned; and even that would be pushing it unless the environment was extraordinarily fruitful and benign. And seven or eight years is an extraordinarily long time for a growing human child to survive alone in a dangerous or even neutral environment.

(ii) The availability of an adult with a repertoire of caretaking skills

This other side to the dynamic is clearly essential too, and is influenced by what kind of attachment the adult experienced in the past, and what kinds of mature, adult attachments are present now.

(iii) Propensity to explore the environment

This too is not to be taken for granted. A land animal that just stayed put like a sea anemone would be doomed. The dynamic has to enable the developing child to become a safe-enough explorer, which includes handling potential threats and new and strange situations, which may be interesting, important and attractive as well as menacing, and all of which are challenging in their different ways. Successful exploring requires also safe arrival – somewhere else, and then back to safe territory again, which requires wider sensitivities too, about time, place and atmosphere as well as orientation in space. It is important which ways are up and down when there is a need to climb trees; Mark Johnson (1987), writing about the relationships between mind, body and activity, discusses orientation in relation to body image, metaphor and projection into 'upness' and 'downness'.

> We grasp (the) structure of verticality repeatedly in thousands of perceptions and activities we experience every day, such as perceiving a tree, our felt sense of standing upright, the activity of climbing stairs, forming a mental image of a flagpole, measuring our

children's heights and experiencing the level of water rising in the bathtub. (Johnson 1987)

We need to think about what we do and how it connects with our organic existence on the one hand and language and metaphor on the other with the same attention to detail neuroscientists and psychoanalysts, for example, apply to their fields. This would make more real the actual nature of every step of the fine-tuning we have gone through since our protozoan times, and is at the level of complexity required to conceptualise consciousness.

(iv) Construction of an internal working image of the outside world

This may be conceived of as, at least, a topographical map – e.g. 'Where did I leave mother (or child)? Which is the way "away" and the way back?'. We should add affect and cognition to other necessary requirements of this aspect of the map, colouring it in as it were. 'Do I recognise mother? What do I see in her? What are the pros and cons of exploring versus returning to her? Whatever I do, how does that feel? If I ignore the parent will I feel guilt? And then what?' These 'basics below the basics' require special stretches of the imagination and often the new use of language, which is why the fundamental biological–philosophical exploration of this area by Jaques Lacan (*see* p. 157) represents yet another subject, characteristically regarded as brilliant by some and nonsense by others. In such areas we really are on the outer edge of the familiar universe.

Bowlby's work is detailed on all aspects of this dynamic system (Bowlby 1969, 1973, 1979) but there are two aspects I want to emphasise – exploratory behaviour, and the elaboration of an internal model or map of the outside world. I was curious whether we could add internal exploration to the developing individual's propensity to explore, but John Bowlby thought this stretched the model too far, taking it into a realm of psychic functioning that required other, traditional models like Freud's. However, for the purposes of a conceptual model for the emergence of consciousness, I want to propose the notion of internal exploration, involving reflection and coming to terms with ideas and feelings, some of which may be unwelcome, as well as external exploration in the physical world.

This complex inner imagery, 'coloured in' by complex and sometimes competing feelings (e.g. about feeling protected or overprotected), supplemented by memory (what last time was like), and spurred by fantasies and anticipations (what if?), is all part of the equipment that enabled proto-humans to live by their wits. This dawning inner imagery, far more elaborate than a simple picture or map, is shaped up by evolution if the species is to have descendants who, as a result, carry the neural framework for the possibility of such imagery in the head. A psychoanalyst might call the beneficial aspects of this the 'introjected good parent'. Someone else, spurning such metaphors, might call it 'backbone'. Either way, the environmental experience has become incorporated; literally (*see* Figure 5.6).

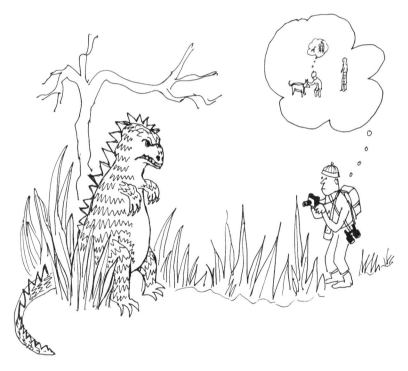

Figure 5.6 The confident explorer

The adult attachment dynamic

Attachment theory began as an exploration of the survival of primate infants and of their emotional development. It is relevant, however, as pointed out above, to adolescent and adult development and group behaviour too. I have mentioned in several contexts the notion of 'regression' – moving back to an earlier, less mature form of behaviour, when under stress.

Like many dynamic processes in psychology, however, the stress doesn't have to be great, or even abnormal. Imagine anyone – an adult – trying anything new and difficult: a first driving or swimming lesson, early steps on stage, preparation for dangerous work in the military or the police or as a schoolteacher in Britain, or just about anything you care to think of. It is not 'childish' to be apprehensive as well as optimistic, or to balance feelings of dependence on a teacher against the wish to proceed independently as soon as possible. This balance includes, I would say, a balance between internal exploration of fears, fantasies and sources of confidence as well as external exploration – reality testing – of the size of the task and the balance between real and imagined dangers. A good teacher or leader gets the balance just right between protection and overprotection, between managing the trainees' anxieties and leaving them to manage on their own, and between showing them what to do and enabling them to find out for themselves. I suggest the equivalent also goes on emotionally and intellectually when people initially doubtful about something new (a theory; a form of art or drama) eventually come to accept it – or indeed reject it for mature reasons. This too contributes to what we make of unfamiliar or uncomfortable ideas – especially new ideas for which we don't have an available 'space'.

In summary: The attachment dynamic enables three necessities for survival and reproduction in proto-humans and humans: (a) adequate care in infancy balanced against (b) the enabling of safe exploratory behaviour and (c) the development of a working 'map' of the world. As mature attachment it continues throughout life, not only in terms of relationships but in the way it is constantly modulated by, and affects, inner feelings and fantasies, in this way contributing to the form and content of consciousness and its unconscious underpinnings. It operates like a guidance system, not always a coherent or consistent one, in the exploration of the individual's intellectual and emotional as well as topographic environment. 'Don't even go there', people say of ideas as well as places. This sense of what is appropriate or sensible for given circumstances is very finely tuned, for example in assessing a 'gut feeling' about real and imagined risks. Approached by a stranger in the street who is asking the time or the way, we rapidly scan an impressive list of judgements, prejudices, memories, scraps of advice, alternative ways of responding, before deciding, in a split second, how to respond. It is said that people meeting socially size each other up (or attempt to) at very high speed in terms of their respective social status, perhaps not so much to avoid danger as embarrassment, something which people sometimes say they would 'rather die' than face. Referring to the 'three-level' way in which we develop and operate, one may see in the nature of such situations and our response to them evolutionary necessities about dealing with strangers, developmental characteristics (what we have learned by experience or been taught by others) and how, given our personality, mood and attitudes at the time of the event, we react to events. For most reasonably competent people, it is as if they carry within themselves a kind of good parent or inner tutor – incorporated by the attachment dynamic into their repertoire of feelings and behaviour, or introjected, as the psychoanalysts would say. But how good does 'good' have to be? 'Good enough' was the recommendation of the distinguished paediatrician-psychoanalyst Donald Winnicott (1972).

The picture that I hope is emerging is of the protozoan necessity to move between favourable and unfavourable environments being now represented in our infinitely more complex lives as sophisticated guidance systems put in place by the relationships and feelings involved in the attachment dynamic; itself an absolute necessity because of the hopelessness of the human infant's chances of survival without caretaking relationships being in place. Lest this seems stretching the point too much, i.e. between an amoeba and ourselves, I suggest that an engineer-philosopher could see the continuity between, say, a submarine and a protozoan, or a modern airliner's flaps and landing gear and the structure and functioning of a bird's wings and legs. The modern human being has state-of-the-art internal wiring for making fine and intuitive judgements about risk versus safety, whether the danger is physical, psychological, cultural or social. For a wider account of evolutionary adaptation and the emerging human mind see Slavin and Kriegman (1992) and Barkow *et al.* (1992).

A burden as a small price for an opportunity

The new brain produced a quite new type of problem for the kind of animal – one might call it a pre-human or proto-human – for whom awareness in two directions (of others, and of self) became super-imposed on raw feelings and impulses. Violent and impulsive killing of a perceived enemy, or uninvited sex with a weaker person, is one thing; something like empathy and conscience is another. Moreover, the emerging complexity of such mixed feelings could have enormously amplified the feelings involved, for example if a surge of adrenalin and a primitive sense of something achieved was 'coloured in' by the newly acquired palette of emotions in such powerful feelings as triumph or guilt. This would be quite a lot for a proto-human to handle; some might have become inhibited from swift action, and risked being killed or injured in return, failed to mate, or gone mad. Those who could handle such muddled and powerful inner feelings, including new inhibitions, yet had no less of a jungle-like existence to contend with, would be likely to become relatively successful in surviving, mating and perhaps even leading in the group. Yet there would have been an explosion of new moods, anxieties, fantasies and baffled wonderings.

No wonder William Golding, in his novel *The Inheritors* about a Neanderthal group (1955), described baffled discovery as a recurring feeling, or that Jack London, in *Before Adam* (1908), described his protagonist ape as being in a constant state of anxiety, which is consistent with recent views of early man (*Australopithecus afarensis*) as more hunted than hunter (Sussman 2006). As we have seen, an even earlier best seller had Nature, or God, announcing a vast loss for humanity as the price of eating from the Tree of Knowledge, despite the smooth words to Eve of the serpent.

From attachment to archetype

I have tried to show the evolution of social and cultural behaviour through the attachment dynamic that equipped us with a cluster of social instincts which enabled, among many other things, awareness and reflecting on inner feelings about external events as part of the developing inner map of the individual's world. If this internal/externally-monitoring system works, enabling those who possess it to maintain intellectual and emotional competence well enough in an increasingly complex and sometimes dangerous world, it would not be surprising if those best-equipped with the kinds of brains to contain and manage such instinctual capacities were more likely to have surviving descendants; that is, ourselves. I suggest that this internal and external monitoring system is essentially a proto-image (it does not have to be a vivid visual image) *of ourselves operating in real, imagined or potential worlds* and *this* is the beginning of an archetype: an inherited potential image of 'what may happen/not happen to me', forged through a million or two years of evolutionary imperatives operating on living experience. Thus we recognise, or think we recognise, friends, enemies, monsters, *et al*. There may have been good reasons to be born with the neural network that could recognise a snake.

But how to operate such a fluid, kaleidoscopic system of ever-changing internal imagery of the inner world of ideas and feelings in relation to the outside world? Some reasonable degree of consistency would be advantageous (given that humanity and human environments are inconsistent and sometime verging on the chaotic) – it would help, in other words, if at the centre of all this input was some kind of editor to check that what the individual felt this morning about a stranger bringing unfamiliar fruits and seeds (possibly life-saving, possibly poisonous) was consistent with the judgement made an hour or so later – memory plus recognition of significance. Something that could take animal-like gut reactions and relate them successfully to external social and cultural demands, juggling all this emotional and perceptual data, and make something (Greek – *poesis*) of it, balancing self-interest, self-esteem and Realpolitik, could represent the beginnings of an observing 'I' at the crossroads of all this information. How this could happen, neuropsychologically, is discussed in Chapter 9. This proto-Ego, or Io, operating in this way, would give its owner the edge when it came to telling useful stories about the world to one's self (the beginning of autobiography and self-identity) as well as to others and making decisions that worked; he or she would be likely to become the first in a line of leaders, priests, magicians, kings and queens or soldiers – he or she who could make acceptable sense of the world, one's role in it, and how to operate in it. By the time such a dominant individual emerged, the group's members – potential leaders and led – could possess within themselves the neural basis or archetype of a 'good-enough' leader. So when, using some kind of primitive language or signing or symbolism, such roles were agreed, minds would have become hard-wired to speak to minds about it, minds that were wired for reception. And reproductive capacity tended to go with such dominance.

The attachment dynamic contributes to the emergence of consciousness in three main ways. First, it connects an evolutionary imperative with both relationships and feelings about relationships. Second, because of the vital importance of group relationships, it shows how cognitive and emotional intelligence applied to internal images of the outside world is as likely to be subject to evolutionary influences as any other set of adaptive instincts. Third, given the inevitability of growing complexity in human relationships (e.g. divided loyalties about contending leaders, friends, enemies and mates, ambivalent feelings about submitting or seeking to be assertive, etc.), there would be an advantage in all these crossed wires coming together and being coordinated in some way within and without, which would require memory, imagination, empathy and anticipation. Conceivably this may be one way for awareness (potential consciousness) to develop its two-way connection (-C-) with 'consciousness by' and 'consciousness of' (*see* pp. 15, 32). These three-dimensional, affect-laden neural networks, containing the physiological possibility of imagination, fantasy and empathy, represent the advanced version of animals' simple representations of the outside world, and for the socio-cultural reasons given are just as essential for survival. *They are imprints of the outside world on the inside world, 'printed' outside again as language, projections and art.* They are archetypes.

We may use them, either acting with their guidance or attributing them to other people, all our lives. To take one example: the violent, risk-taking, manipulative, impulsive villain or hero is one of the *dramatis personae* people might have in their repertoire, either minimally (at one end of the spectrum of possibilities) such that it would never be elicited except perhaps in fantasy or if ill, intoxicated or acting (or writing a convincing crime story?) while at the other end of the spectrum it could be so near the surface, so readily provoked, that its possessor is labelled as a psychopath or as 'disturbed' in some other way, or in some special circumstances as heroic. Archetypes interact with the culture because they are so universal that like Genet's real or imaginary (actually, both) Bishop, Judge and General (*see* p. 99) the culture generates them as well as recognises them. We 'know' (recognise) such roles before they emerge and acknowledge them when they do.

From innate predispositions to culture

A short diversion from archetypes to other neuropsychological pre-dispositions illustrates other examples of the primarily neural inter-acting with the prevailing culture. That pattern of feeling, cognition, anomalous language development and behaviour identified now as autistic spectrum disorder can demonstrate two phenomena: how a disabling condition can nevertheless persist down the generations, and how it may help shape a culture and become an advantage within it. People identified as on the autistic spectrum of disorder are from childhood less good at handling feelings, empathy, developing what is known as a theory of other people's minds and less skilled at the emotional side of attachment. Possibly they resemble one kind of child left behind by our ancestors. Yet whatever may be the genetic component of the condition is still with us, and demonstrates that like most things attachment isn't 'all or none' every time but a balance of probabilities. Thus there persist in the genetics of our nervous systems patterns for thinking, feeling and behaviour that can be expressed in quite different ways depending on the socio-cultural conditions. Thus, human parents are adaptable enough to love and care for infants who are less obviously or immediately rewarding and responsive than infants are ordinarily expected to be: this is part of the adaptability, empathy and imaginativeness that makes us human. Also, a 'disad-vantage' in one epoch or situation may be advantageous in another. If there were autistic-like children among our ancestors, there may also have been enough mothers able to make special allowances for them, and love and nurture them.

Taking autistic spectrum characteristics as the example, Simon Baron-Cohen (2003) has pointed out the potential advantage for a computer-based, high-technology culture of the autistic spectrum qualities of highly focused and systematic ways of functioning, es-pecially when allied to high intelligence of an objective, organising kind. As a set of dispositions that are currently highly valued and lead to industrial and academic developments, this is likely to enable economic and social success, marriage and child-rearing in a popu-lation group who, on balance, might have had less such encourage-ment in other periods. As with the earlier example, what may be regarded as a disadvantage or eccentricity in one cultural setting or period, or even a clinically-labelled condition, in another time and place *contributes to* the culture. In Baron-Cohen's account he widens the notion of autism to being an example of the extreme male mind, and its current cultural and technological contributions may account for at least some of the apparent increase in some populations of autistic spectrum personality.

This is not the place to argue the pros and cons of this position, but I find it intriguing. It provides a model that puts 'clinical disorder', indeed any kind of disability, into another perspective. Later we will see that the same can be said of most 'psychiatric' categories, though without denying that they can also be distressing and disabling. We can therefore consider the parts such experiences and behaviour patterns play in consciousness without being distracted by consider-ations of 'normal' and 'abnormal' consciousness; such categorisation is useful in clinical circumstances, but is less helpful when trying to consider the full biological and psychological picture.

It also suggests human potentialities, a vast array of them, being laid down in the human genome like fine wines, awaiting the moment when a special cast of mind recognises a special kind of cultural need, and fulfils it. It is one of the ways arts and sciences and ways of organising ourselves move forward. Our genes are full of silent regions – one may wonder what other capabilities and ideas are written down in that vast bible of recipes, awaiting the right moment for their cultural expression. Do prophets, visionaries and some science-fiction writers have intuitive access to this neurally-based, ultimately genetic pool of knowledge?

How does culture get into the mind?

Again, I am anticipating future chapters, particularly 7 and 8, and summarising some of what has gone before, but wanted to mention at this point how each turn of the brain–culture cycle is completed – i.e. how culture 'gets in' – so that I can use it as a kind of grappling hook to project across Chapter 6 and to the two that follow.

By 'culture' I hope it will be clear by now that I do not mean only the 'big' culture of big important people and institutions (though this is by no means excluded) but rather the whole made and commercial environment, including its prevailing customs, attitudes and behav-iour patterns along with all its artefacts and embellishments – all the memes. You might say that all this stuff, from junk to genius, is simply 'out there', observed and recorded or ignored, by an observing brain, on which the external culture writes as if on a blank slate. The 'blank slate' theory assumes that we are born with no significant social or cultural predispositions, and that for every individual it is acquired anew from outside. The model for the mind I am developing in this book depends on a continuous and complex cycling between the developing mind 'within' and the developing culture 'outside' that the mind itself uses, develops and elaborates. This external product of the mind then hauls the mind forward in its development – hence the grappling hook analogy. The 'grappling hook' is made of imagery, symbolism, language and metaphor. It could be conceptualised as a kind of psychological DNA making crucial connections between brain and culture. If the reader has a sense of what is meant by mother-figure, or father-figure, or monster (that is, if the curious black ink-marks on this page light up images of these in the neural network behind the eyes, a minor miracle if ever there was one), that is because the wiring for them is already there in the brain.

Years of hearing or reading about such archetypes or seeing them again and again in books, drama or films may have reinforced and embellished them; but (so my argument goes) the rudimentary circuits, the building blocks, are part of the structure of the nervous system, because during our evolution those who had the kinds of brain best-wired to recognising mothers, fathers or monsters had the evolutionary edge over those less well-endowed. The former kinds of brains were more likely to be replicated down the ages; this is an important quality of the evolution of the brain, but its importance is in millions of small ways rather than representing a gigantic, astonishing step. There is nothing extraordinary in an infant recognising a mother image and responding to maternal handling, any more than it is extraordinary that the infant can metabolise oxygen, water, fat, carbohydrate and protein and make use of warmth. Both, the nutrition and the image-construction, are literally vital (i.e. enable survival), and so much part of our being that the existence of the necessary processes tends to be taken for granted unless they go wrong. But they should not be taken for granted if we want to understand the emergence of self; the anatomy and physiology for taking in, digesting and using nutrition, and the corresponding physical capacity to recognise and respond to caretaking adults, which is the beginning of the capacity to recognise and respond to the world, is evolved into us as constituents of self. But the imagery that is the necessary part of recognising the outside world gets 'fixed' by memory (as a photograph is fixed by chemicals) and then elaborated by fantasy, imagination and anticipation (forward projection of memory and fantasy), with qualities attributed to the outside world – some of them there, and some of them not there. This is the first spark of what becomes consciousness, and then the beginnings of self-consciousness.

If we didn't have the kind of brain able to take 'mother' (*et al.*) in with the milk and hold that image in the head, and colour in the image with feelings, and then attribute this inner picture to the world outside – i.e. project it out again to use 'outside' – neither we nor the culture with which we surround ourselves would ever have got started.

Twists in the tale

Histories and mysteries: philosophies of mind and the uncertain nature of reality

'The body makes the mind'

'The Body', said John Donne (1572–1631), 'makes the minde, not that it created it a minde, but forms it a good or bad minde; and this minde may be confounded with soul without any injustice to reason or philosophy; then the soul is enabled by the body, not the body by the soul; my body licences my soul to see the world's beauties through mine eyes; to hear pleasant things through mine ears, and affords it apt organs for the convenience of all perceivable delight.' Donne, a poet and divine, and Dean of St Paul's, led a full and lively life (one may deduce from his poetry the full range of the 'apt organs' he refers to), and at one point was thrown into prison. He wrote the above words in his 'Paradoxes and Problems' around 1590 (Hayward 1929).

It would have been interesting to know what Donne would have made of Benedict Spinoza (1632–1677), a Dutch-Jewish philosopher and student of optics and astronomy who was excommunicated for his supposed pantheism and atheism, then regarded by the religious authorities as one and the same thing. Spinoza described Mind (thought) as one of the attributes of God, the only other attribute knowable to Man being 'extension', or things, including the material body. It may seem a fine point, but in that he saw mind and matter coming from the same source, he was not speaking as a dualist like René Descartes (1596–1650), for whom mind and body represented two fundamentally distinct phenomena. Thus Descartes is the philosopher most associated with the philosophy of dualism, and just about everyone else with monism, or the belief that everything in the universe – mind or spirit and things – comes from a single source, be that source God or Nature. (*See* John Searle on this, below.) Spinoza regarded God and Nature being the same, and the source of both the mind (thought) and extension (things), which has been described as essentially a monist i.e. single-source philosophy. The pros and cons of dualism have dogged studies of consciousness ever since (and indeed before the distinction was formulated). Most of the modern neuroscientific literature on consciousness is monist, i.e. it assumes that the mind and consciousness are, indeed can only be, products of the physical brain. As Dennett (1991), one of the leading modern philosophers of consciousness, puts it:

> *Dualism, the view that minds are composed of some non-physical and utterly mysterious stuff; and vitalism, the view that living things contain some special physical but equally mysterious stuff – élan vital, have been relegated to the trash heap of history, along with alchemy and astrology. (Dennett 1991)*

However, by discarding the concept of dualism Dennett may have thrown out some of the real and relevant stuff with the rubbish, as we shall see, because this approach risks not taking a full account of all of the world outside the brain too.

Searle (1997), in his excellent review of the work of several of the key modern explorers of consciousness, provides a useful service in clarifying what one might call degrees of dualism. Dualists, he suggests, divide into 'substance dualists' who think mind and body are completely separate, and 'property dualists' who see the possibility of 'mental' and 'physical', although quite different, representing two distinct properties of the human being. Monists, however, divide into idealists, who see everything as ultimately mental, and materialists who think that everything, including what we label 'mental', as being ultimately physical (*see* Figure 6.1). Writing in 1997, Searle makes the interesting observation that most people in our civilisation accept some kind of dualism, believing themselves to have both a mind (or soul) and a body, while the great majority of philosophy, psychology, cognitive science, neurobiology and artificial intelligence scientists and academics are essentially materialistic monists, seeing no other perspective consistent with contemporary science. But Searle identifies a problem for them: 'once you have described all the material facts in the world, you still seem to have a lot of mental phenomena left over', which materialists deal with by reducing mental facts to material phenomena or by denying that they exist at all. 'The history of the philosophy of mind over the past one hundred years has been in large part an attempt to get rid of the mental by showing that no

mental phenomena exist over and above physical phenomena'
(Searle 1997).

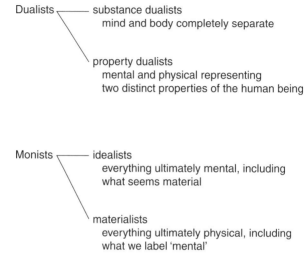

Figure 6.1   Dualists and monists

Memory and the body

Closely linked with questions of mind and body is the notion, prominent in the nineteenth century, that memory was inherited along
with the physical characteristics of forebears. The name most associated with the inheritance of acquired (physical) characteristics is
Jean-Baptiste de Lamarck (1744–1829). Although abandoned and
discredited, Lamarck's more general views about evolution make him
one of its notable pioneers; but nevertheless the idea that a trait
acquired in life (such as the blacksmith's large muscles) could reappear in his offspring is not thought entirely compatible with current
views of what genes do. The debate about the possibility of Lamarckian
inheritance continues (for example Fine 1979; Steele *et al.* 1998) and
as serious a biological commentator as Stephen Jay Gould has argued
that, while there is no definite evidence that cells, presumably via
their cellular RNA (ribonucleic acid), can transcript experience into
DNA (deoxyribonucleic acid), Lamarckism does provide a conceptual
model for the kind of non-chemical, environmental evolution of

behavioural innovation (Gould 1989), which is the concept I employed earlier for shaping populations in the direction of using and being able to use attachment behaviour and which represents a form of cultural evolution. Nevertheless, as far as evolution in the genes is concerned, Darwinism is about selection, by evolutionary necessity, of random variation in the genetic makeup of species – random not in a strictly mathematical sense, but meaning simply not directed to any particular adaptation; it is that which works which survives. Lamarckism, however, was a theory of directed variation, a particular variation acquired in its lifetime being bequeathed to its offspring. Most people do not accept that there is yet any convincing evidence for a route from experience in an animal's lifetime via its DNA to pass on to its descendants; and yet the idea of goal-directed genetic design has been a spur to some agnostics and atheists who, while not accepting creationism as an act of faith, believe that there has simply not been enough time for the extraordinary fine-tuning of living things to their environments to have happened by chance, especially when two or three adaptations have seemed to be needed concurrently, rather than in a series in which each builds upon the previous change. Lamarckism, as a model for directed adaptation which might prove compatible with things yet to be discovered about genes and immune systems, will not quite go away, and seems to remain on the back-burner of evolutionary theory for thoughtful Darwinians.

The only reference to Lamarckism I can find in my row of Richard Dawkins' books is in one of his earlier works (1982), in which after – to be fair – a debate that he extends over 14 closely argued pages, he concludes that:

> *few things would more devastate my world view than a demonstrated need to return to the theory of evolution that is traditionally attributed to Lamarck. It is one of the few contingencies for which I might offer to eat my hat. (Dawkins 1982)*

To be accurate, Dawkins begins his account with these words, but does repeat his offer, and refines his argument to affirm that his hat really is tough and distasteful. (Has he nibbled at it before?) I could not find Lamarck mentioned again, so perhaps he is not anxious to set this particular hare running. Nevertheless Dawkins' position is a heroic one, and his critique of Lamarckian ideas (Dawkins 1982) is worth reading. Having said that, I do think his wager is sufficiently carefully worded to make the need to stew his hat unlikely.

Pinker (1997), a cognitive psychologist who sees language as an inherited instinct, dismisses the idea of cultural evolution on the grounds that (a) the premise of cultural evolution is that it is 'directed' by a single phenomenon such as 'the march of progress' or 'the ascent of man', (b) that it is close to the notion of the spread of memes, (c) that it requires a Lamarckian (i.e. discredited) model, and (d) having set Lamarck up, Pinker says this means that no one has any idea how cultural evolution might work. For Pinker, clearly cultural evolution is a no-go area. However, none of these assertions about it are correct.

My own instinct is that we haven't heard the last of Lamarckism. Meanwhile, my own proposal for the inheritance of patterns of feeling, imagery and behaving is through the route of those inherited (i.e. genetically loaded) neurobiological characteristics favoured by the cultural environment, which, for reasons I have explained, are as powerfully influential for crucial aspects of human development as the physical or chemical environment. Also for the future, we do not yet know all that intracellular microtubules – potentially micro nervous systems (*see* pp. 149,185) might do within the cell.

Other ways in which body and memory interact have been described, for example by Rosenfield (1993) who argues also for the connectedness between the flow of perception, the sense of body image and a sense of time and space which lock memory and consciousness together inseparably. Like Edelman (1989) he would say 'no consciousness without memory'.

Laura Otis (1994) has given an account of memory from the more historical, literary and cultural perspectives (*see* p. 164), filling out more of the cultural side of the mind–culture interaction, while Levin (1985) in a work I found complex but poetic incorporates conceptions of the human body with bodies of knowledge in an intriguing dance of actuality and metaphors. 'The wholeness of our being takes place as much in the life of our feet and hands and eyes as it does in our head, our brains and our "mind"', with which I think many neurologists would agree.

Cultural evolution: summary

What I would like to extract for the notion of cultural evolution as a connecting-rod in my model of consciousness is a kind of para-Lamarckism. The dramatic growth and development during the evolution of the human brain and (a) the consequent need for the human infant to be born while still small (to get through the birth canal) and thus still biologically premature, (b) a further consequent and imperative need for close and effective attachment to others and (c) its new cognitive and affective potential would all be likely to vary from individual to individual. Some brains would be more effective than others as integrators, recorders and organisers of the new cognitive and emotional data from the outside world and from within, and able to take advantage of the protection and care of the attachment dynamic, their neural wiring being better at it. Metaphorically, those kinds of brains were better 'studios' for handling the drama and the news from the outside world and the opportunities within it. What was inherited and became innate was not the drama and the news, but the 'studios' and their neural equipment. Thus they had the ability to reproduce cultural impressions – archetypes – from this inherited machinery. Thus, not the actual programmes but dedicated though adaptable production equipment became innate.

The mind makes the world

Much of the cognitive psychological and neuropsychological literature works like this. On the one hand we have the world spinning along in its own peculiar way, moderately well known as far as its history, sliding tectonic plates and the rise and fall of civilisations are concerned. Not all known, but eminently knowable. And over here (and I have to say I'm back in the fairground among the carousels again) someone is setting up his stall, all circuits and flickering bulbs, to show how the brain observes and becomes conscious of the world.

Now, I don't want to become embroiled with Bishop George Berkeley and his view that the world is no more than a product of the mind; but just as John Donne, if I understand his somewhat archaic words correctly, said not only that the body creates the mind 'but forms it a good or bad minde', I would say that the mind doesn't make the world but does shape it up in a way that not only suits us, but enables it to be comprehensible, even visible, to us. We shape it, in a sense, in our own preferred image. To look at this argument, we need to leave the world of neuroscience and psychology, and to pay attention to two very different groups: social philosophers, especially of the 'postmodern' schools, and the more thoughtful political scientists on the one hand; and quantum physicists on the other. But first, because among our fantasies is the notion that physicists are *real* scientists and on firmer ground, we will begin with them.

The mind makes reality: physicists' perspectives

The bedrock of science as opposed to art is supposedly its objectivity; but the bedrock is on the slide for important areas of science. In the classical physics of nineteenth-century science (the kind of 'objectivity' that preoccupies and distracts whole swathes of contemporary psychology and psychiatry) the observer can remain detached from what is being described, categorised and measured. This science is still enormously important – it is how engineers can design bridges that stay up. But in quantum mechanics, which actually works experimentally and in nuclear technology, there is evidence that at other levels of understanding the world and its structure is inseparable from the process of observing and measuring it. For example, observing what subatomic particles do affects what they do (*see* Schrödinger's mysterious cat, below). This is significant, bearing in mind that there are psychologists and psychiatrists who are convinced that an interviewer can make a purely objective assessment in an interview.

As stated in the most general terms (as the anthropic principle) by Barrow and Tipler (1986) our human existence imposes a stringent selection effect upon the type of universe we could expect to observe. This requires a particular set of physical qualities in the natural universe to exist in order that a particular kind of consciousness could come into being that can even begin to comprehend it. This, I think, is consistent conceptually with the notion of archetypal predispositions to perceive the world in a certain way. Thus, the brain may not *make* the material universe, but our particular universe is one in which a very particular kind of brain is able to evolve and this kind of brain is able to see (and measure) a particular perspective of the universe. We are, so to speak, locked into a universe we cannot really be detached from for the sake of pursuing 'objectivity'. I believe this has echoes not only of the neurological points made on pages 1 and 28, but of Spinoza's position too. It is worth reading what Barrow and Tipler (1986), Barrow (1995) and Davies (1982, 1992 and Davies and Brown 1986) say about all this; their work is referred to again in Chapter 11. But this whole line of thinking, complex though it is, says something useful about consciousness, challenging the notion of consciousness as something primarily to do with what goes on inside the box – our skulls – and its wiring. In some way, which I will return to from time to time in the rest of the book as a dog worries a bone, the anthropic principle is not about 'only the mind being real' or 'only the material world being real', but that the one is adapted to the other; that aspects of the material world have shaped a particular kind of mind that can sense and observe it. Correspondingly, the unknowable that lies outside this cosy relationship is possible. This theme is taken up again in Chapters 9 and 11.

Schrödinger's mysterious cat

Erwin Schrödinger (1887–1961) was a most distinguished Austrian physicist who, in his classic essay *What is Life?* (1944) anticipated the discovery of genes. His thought-experiment with the cat (not of course a real pussy) sought to illustrate, curiously, not something only about physics but something about consciousness. The idea of the experiment was that the imaginary cat in an imaginary sealed box is subject to the completely unpredictable emission of a particle – which, if emitted, would release gas which killed the cat. But since the box is sealed, and the particle's emission is completely unpredictable, not only do we not know whether the cat is alive or dead but the 'actual' imagined cat is 'in reality' neither alive nor dead, until the box is opened and the cat examined.

I have often had it explained to me by physicists that this thought-experiment illustrated something about particle physics, which is how it is often presented in the literature, but Pagels' account (1982) suggests that Schrödinger intended to demonstrate how *crazy* was the notion that the whole world was as unpredictable as the activities of particles, or that the material universe could not exist independently of our observations of it. Schrödinger, rather, maintained that the famous bizarreness of particle behaviour (e.g. being in two different places at the same time) was confined to the quantum world only.

This experiment has been described many times as if demonstrating something about the uncertainty of the physical world. When I have tried to challenge physicists to explain why it doesn't merely demonstrate psychological uncertainty (i.e. we don't know whether the cat is alive or dead) I have received only glazed and (I think) pitying glances. Not until I came across Pagels' account did I realise that Schrödinger was being – I think – ironic about the notion that until there is consciousness of reality there is no material reality: George Berkeley again. Elsewhere he was still clearer, stating that we must distinguish between physical indeterminacy and human consciousness (Schrödinger 1957). So there you are, and I mention it here because it is a thought-experiment widely portrayed as a demonstration of uncertainty in physics when it is really about consciousness. But you will find many subtly different accounts of the cat, the particle and the box and what it is all about. Meanwhile, as Schrödinger himself might (possibly) have said, enough already about the cat.

Plato's cave

I have never thought that the classical fable of the pre-eminent Greek philosopher Plato (427–347 BC) about the prisoner in the cave conveyed all that much, but perhaps that is because one of his central tenets, that things aren't as they seem, has long become part of our cultural inheritance. He refers to the kind of education citizens of the ideal state would receive, before which they are like prisoners in a cave, observing only shadows cast from the outside world. Once released into the sunlight they are able to return to see things for what they really are. The catch is that the State described in Plato's *Republic* is very strictly regulated, even to the kind of poetry permitted, and the prisoners' eventual 'illumination' may be more doctrinal than a step nearer wider truths. But Plato was most interesting, I think, in other areas, and described something very close to archetypes nearly 2000 years before a very similar concept emerged as a central tenet of Jung's psychology. This is discussed in Chapter 7.

Other alternative realities

Postmodernism, a term which after some research I have concluded means 'next' (like the fashion store) as much as it means anything, refers to a cluster of attitudes and thinking which include moral relativism, multiple alternative views of perceived 'realities', and truths and meanings being provisional rather than established. Again, that things aren't what they seem; in which respect psychoanalysis must have been among one of the oldest modern postmodern schools, as also perhaps were the surrealists. Magritte's painting of a pipe, entitled 'Ceci n'est pas une pipe', is an example, and one may suggest lugubriously, as befits the purposes of a book on consciousness, that this kind of thing is also a '*joke*', and that we should not forget wit and humour as a kind of solvent where alternative realities are juxtaposed and need to be brought together and mixed into ambiguities, for example in telling jokes about things which make us angry or scared.

The history of the newspaper cartoon, like much of drama, and despite being associated with 'being funny', is characteristically about combining humour with seriousness and sometimes tragedy. People say, as a kind of ethical gold standard, that you couldn't be funny about the Holocaust, or any other genocide, which I think is true, yet newspaper cartoons about the horrors of war, mass murder, mass neglect and starvation are perfectly feasible and in the first and second world wars, for example, there were cartoons which helped shape consciousness.

Jean Genet's play *The Balcony* (1957) nicely captures the sceptical questioning of what we take for granted. A Chief of Police is trying to find a way to restore order in a city-state which is fast descending into chaos and anarchy, its leaders having fled. He confides his fears to his friend, the madame of a brothel. She tells him that even as they speak she has three of her regulars in. One of the men is dressed up as a Bishop, another as a Judge and the third as a General, the better, as one might put it, to share their fantasies with her girls. The Police Chief requisitions them to join him on the balcony of the brothel, where they nod and wave to the roaring crowd as he delivers a passionate plea for the restoration of order; he then drives the three around the city in an open car. The angry shouting of the crowd turns into cheers and order is restored. They were hardly 'pretending' to be leaders of the Church, the Law and the Army; they didn't need to, because what mattered was the image of these three forms of authority. But to what extent is a 'real' Bishop, Judge or General a man dressed up for these roles? (In Alan Bennett's play, *The Madness of King George*, the King corrects a courtier who was busy reassuring anxious visitors by saying that the King was not 'himself' today, with the observation that he had forgotten how to *seem*.)

There is a whole stratum in recent literary, social and political criticism which questions assumptions about the nature of reality, some of its principles discussed in Berger's and Luckman's *The Social Construction of Reality* (1967) and in clinical terms by Laing (1967). It is too vast a body of commentary to review here, though I will mention the philosophers Jean Baudrillard (e.g. Gane 1991; Kellner 1995), Barthes (Barthes 1973, 1977) and Derrida (Wood 1992) as three ways into the subject. Some of the writing and concepts are nearly incomprehensible, though I find Barthes more accessible; but one may, if one is inclined, sympathise, because like both the psychoanalysts and the quantum physicists (e.g. Bohr 1963; Bohm 1974, 1980) they are trying to describe concepts which are so different from the norm, so much at the edge or over the edge of everyday experience and assumptions, that they have to invent new languages, new metaphors and new imagery to convey what they are trying to say. Indeed, some of this modern (or 'postmodern') philosophy is about language itself, and about other cultural signs and symbols (semiology – ways we signal to each other), for example in Barthes (1973). Not surprisingly, much of it is highly acclaimed on the one hand and derided or ignored on the other, but it is, I think, an important field in the study of consciousness, since that which is taken for granted in the culture, and that which challenges what is taken for granted, between them modulate what our minds take in.

From the perspective of this book, the issue is not who is 'right', radical philosopher-political activist or conservative, rather that there have always been alternative versions of reality available, more than anyone can attend to on any given moment or in a lifetime, and much human time and energy goes into persuading other people that this lifestyle, that form of art, this philosophy or that political perspective is the 'right' one. One might say that sanity (or, less sharply, normality) represents a cluster of generally socially and culturally acceptable assumptions (hence, common sense) which is a broad path in some truly liberal cultures (though some modern 'liberals' do like to keep breadth of opinion on a tight rein if they can) and decidedly narrow in autocratic, tyrannical and theocratic societies.

At which point I will venture no further into these deep and murky waters, except to say that in their different ways Freud and the post-Freudians, and Marx and the post-Marxists, pursue rather complementary themes. The psychoanalysts' position is that the feelings, attitudes, motivation, behaviour and alliances of their clientele are driven by unconscious influences of which they have little appreciation until they begin to achieve 'insight'. Social radicals maintain that the people are similarly driven by social and cultural pressures, expectations and influences of which they are unaware, until their consciousness or 'awareness' is raised. The psychoanalyst sees the unanalysed client as more or less neurotic; the political activist sees the politically 'unaware' as insufficiently informed and educated. Both schools of thought have their corrective and persuasive methods, as have priests, magicians, myth-makers, story-tellers and soothsayers throughout human history, and we have more than ever of them today. Both represent unconsciousness of a kind, one psychological and the other socio-cultural, and both affect how we may be.

7

Archetype

Two serious heresies: the mystery of the archetype, and the inheritance of experience

What is an archetype?

The idea of archetypes and archetypal forms is controversial and refers to several different though related ideas which are particularly associated with the psychology of Jung (Jacobi 1971). I want to introduce them in this chapter because although there are real differences between different authorities the archetypal hypothesis seems to me to possess important general characteristics which stand up despite the undoubted differences in usage and the details attributed to them. These differences are real, not hair-splitting, as we shall see; although I believe the concept is broad enough to represent a cluster of phenomena, more than one of which may be valid.

Before seeing what different usage is made of the term I want to outline the kind of 'vehicle' for the mind they are; nothing less, I would say, than a set of templates for the mind; a structure, incorporated into the form and function of our nervous systems and which gives shape to the form and function of the way we perceive, feel and think. Apart from being properties of the brain they aren't visible or perceptible, but they shape the mind as surely as, say, the lie, pattern and texture of the land shapes what happens to water falling across it. One may think of them – metaphorically – as a kind of lattice-work or crystalline structure for the mind, not only enabling it to perceive, think and feel, but also *setting limits* on what it may perceive, think or feel, in which they bear a conceptual relationship to the notion of the anthropic principle (*see* p. 96). To jump ahead a little, one could argue that we do not know the unknowable because we do not have the mental equipment to apprehend it, and this limitation is not one of intelligence or brain power – both rather vague concepts, in fact – but with what we are equipped to perceive or think, rather as we are not equipped to smell what a dog smells or hear what a bat hears. To this I would add – though this is one of the sources of dispute – that archetypes are evolved and inherited; they are complex, culturally-connected instincts acquired during the processes of survival just as simpler instincts like 'fright, fight and flight' are. One might say the archetype informs the organism precisely *what* to take fright at, fight or flee from.

This broad notion of archetypes spans three areas fundamental to understanding consciousness, and can be used to make connections between them. These are the evolution of the human mind, the development of the personal psychology of relationships (known in psychodynamic theory as object relationships), and the formation of inner imagery drawn primarily from the outside world though 'coloured' – by which I mean given emotional and narrative power – from within.

Thinking in terms of archetypes may seem surprising to people coming across them for the first time. What is also surprising, and I mention it because throughout this book I have suggested that the politics of academic convention constantly plays cat and mouse with the politics of consciousness (and vice versa), archetypes have been largely disregarded if not discredited in official or correct psychology and psychiatry and in all the recent 'big' studies of consciousness. It is however a coming idea, and as evidence for this I would cite their re-emergence, albeit under other names, in important areas of language studies and neuroscience. I would recommend Jean Knox's recent detailed review of attachment theory in relation to archetypal psychology and its variants (Knox 2003) although she takes a more critical specific view of the idea of archetypes than I do for the purposes of this book, for which I wanted a more general mechanism for the innate incorporation of social experience during evolution.

The archetype as a connection in a model for consciousness

Before coming to different academic views on the nature and properties of archetypes I will illustrate my own version, the one I will be using as a key structure in the model for consciousness I am describing.

Beginning again with the simple, single-celled protozoan, how it operates is relatively simple; simple, that is, for an animal, although infinitely complex compared with, say, drying paint or solidifying cement. It is a one-celled search engine with a limited number of goals; it approaches favourable conditions (water and nutrients in the right temperature range) and avoids unfavourable conditions, not because they are 'naturally favourable' but because the cell comes from a line of organisms that happened to survive in such conditions and are still with us because of what works. This micro-behaviour pattern, as effective as a simple thermostat, is its *modus operandi* (*see* p. 54).

It works, and because it works the protozoan has similar successors with the same inherited *modus operandi*. One might even stretch a point and say that it is not so much that the protozoan 'has' this way of working; rather, this way of working *is* the motor that drives the protozoan and lets it survive, and in its way is every bit as remarkable as the rest of the cell – its nucleus, its semi-permeable membrane that acts as a boundary but lets the necessary substances in and out, its internal metabolism and so on. By unwittingly adapting to its environment – its nutrient culture – it defends and promotes its own inner nutrient culture. Thus what I have called its search engine uses the external nutrient culture to defend and preserve its *inner* nutrient culture – its metabolism – and this, of course, preserves the organism as a whole, including its search engine. It is a neat arrangement. I would describe this *modus operandi* of the protozoan as the simplest kind of archetype: it represents how to make a successful print – a route map if you like – printed (and reprintable) within, with its printer's block shaped by the outside world. Remember that the protozoan doesn't know what it's doing any more than does drying paint or a thermostat. But then our basic proto-archetype is just like the other more sophisticated archetypes we will mention later: they too are beyond consciousness, inaccessible, more neurology than psychology; they are not the 'route maps' themselves, which are guidance systems that grow in each living organism, but the innate, dedicated printing system that makes it possible for the organism to generate them. At the risk of overdoing my explanation of the difference: take a simple reflex, withdrawing from an animal's snapping mouth – we don't inherit the image of a crocodile but we do inherit what it takes to know the shape and movement of what to jump back from plus the hormonal (adrenalin) and neurophysiological and locomotor systems necessary to enable rapid backing off.

A few million years forward, and we may consider the potentially helpless infant who will die if it doesn't have within it the wherewithal as we have seen for attachment behaviour (Chapter 5). It requires a caretaking, parenting adult and the ability to recognise, attract and respond rewardingly to one. One can never know how many false and fortuitous starts helpless infants and potential parents made; given the odds against survival, the time involved and the DNA evidence that hardly a handful of human beings started out from that area of North Africa not far from the myth of the site of Eden, we must assume the successful ones would have been in a minority. A small creature (your remote ancestor and mine) clearly came through this almost unwinnable lottery with the kind of mind that held the capacity for human attachment in its psychological and bodily repertoire; and since in the first tiny minorities of survivors they were chance developments already there and innate, not learned, some of their offspring would have these qualities too. An unimaginable time later we take the loving mother, the gurgling, smiling, gazing baby and the warm, well-provided nursery, indeed a whole child-care culture, for granted. That initially fortuitous, later essential, life-preserving, self-preserving, image-forming, *inner* image-forming (in mother *and* child), iconic cultural relationship represents a basic, biologically-based, evolved archetype.

Even this primate child/parent interaction is a relatively simple archetype, just a little up from the reptile of 300 million years ago that (unconsciously) risks self-sacrifice by hanging around its eggs and looking after them; but that good beast (*see* p. 71), a very indirect ancestor of course, nevertheless bequeathed us some sort of fragment of behaviour pattern, something in the DNA and the reptilian parts of our brains, in the subsequent life stream. Infinitely more elaborate archetypal capacity and behaviour follows.

What else is an archetype?

In general speech the word archetype is used rather like 'stereotype', for example the archetypal rock star, Englishman or retired colonel, usually inaccurately. Etymologically it doesn't mean 'typical', nor time honoured, but the first, or prototype: literally, the first impression, printing or stamp.

The theory of archetypes stands in contrast to the *tabula rasa* idea that the human infant is born with a 'blank slate' of a mind on which future experience writes. It seems unlikely that compared with everything else we are born with, not least a highly complex nervous system which has clearly evolved over so many millions of years, the mind of all things should start out blank each time. It does seem, for example, that we are born with what it takes to learn languages with enormous efficiency (Chomsky 1971; Lyons 1991; Pinker 1994) and, as with archetypes, not with an inner dictionary or phrase book but the neural structures necessary to make connections between words, syntax and symbolic meanings. Chomsky (1971) refers not to archetypes but to 'deep structures' in the brain which are universal and which enable and modulate this learning process. Structural anthropologists like Lévi-Strauss (1967) also believe that there are innate psychological factors which guide how we perceive social relationships.

The idea of archetypes formulated by the Athenian philosopher Plato (428–347 BC), Socrates' pupil, included the idea that the innate 'forms' with which we were born came from an ideal realm beyond our minds but accessible indirectly by the mind, and that they together represent a taxonomy of anything we might in the course of our lives imagine or recognise (= know again). He saw them as universal essential qualities – they might be objects, or qualities like largeness, beauty, justice or the subjective sense of colour which, as with other qualia (personal, subjective experience, like the colour of a tomato), seem impossible to objectify, although Ramachandran and Blakeslee (1998) have boldly tried using a thought-experiment, though not, I think, with success. They are nearer the mark in widening the issue and suggesting that there is a need to reconcile the 'I' view with the third-person view of the universe, which they identify as 'the single most important unsolved problem in science'. With the experience of 'I', the closer you get the more it is somewhere else, in which respect 'I'-ness, I think, has the qualities of qualia, and perhaps of an archetype too. Perhaps Plato was on the right lines, even if his notion has been both set aside in philosophy and psychology if revised or rediscovered over the years. For the moment, let us keep the notions of qualia and archetypal form as sharing something important: the notion of something innate and primary in our brain; and also *pre-imaginative*, because Plato took the view that we could not imagine 'red', or understand the word for 'red', without the Form being there first. These Forms are paradigms of anything we can imagine or perceive in our lives – which is why we can imagine or see what we come across. If such 'forms' don't come from an 'ideal other world', perhaps they come from where archetypes come from – incorporated examples of biological-social developments in individuals that had evolutionary advantage and became innate in the species. But, a point I will take up later, do they therefore represent a world of abstraction, partly ideas, partly cultural and partly neural, yet non-existent in any single one of these three areas? If that was a supportable argument, there is possibly some concordance with the notion of the anthropic principle and aspects of quantum physics, and we *might* be describing a domain of highly influential abstractions which – contrary to what I wrote in the Preface of this book – is neither entirely natural nor supernatural.

The archetypes of the collective unconscious: CG Jung

Jacobi (1968), Stevens (1982, 2002) and Storr (1998) provide first-rate accounts of the analytical psychology of CG Jung, though as with Freud it is worth reading what the man himself wrote. As with Freud, he wrote and taught a vast amount over a long period and much of it now approaching a century ago, and it is not surprising that such work contains changes of mind, changes of direction and inconsistencies. Jung had a special extra problem in that he was writing at the time of the rise of the science and politics of eugenics, with racialism reaching one of its periodic peaks in national socialism, and the idea of the collective unconscious became blurred with highly ethnocentric notions of 'race memories'. To be fair to Jung's critics, some of his ideas about racial memory did at one point seem tied to particular human groups, yet there is more than enough in his writings to see that the idea of the collective unconscious makes most sense psychologically as something common to the whole of humanity.

Where Freud described the individual unconscious, Jung added another: the collective unconscious, the repository of the archetypes, and one way to convey the essence of what it is about is a geological model (*see* Figure 7.1) – mountain peaks representing individuals, each separate most of the way down, and then gradually merging with the foothills of other mountains and then with the whole underlying geology of the world representing the collective experience of the human race, which to me means that we are all born with broadly the same kinds of brains. The experience of finding that people across the world have great individual differences as people, differences as groups and cultures, but have very similar feelings and attitudes to everyone else not far below the surface is a common one. Many things confirm that the human race is uniracial below its multicultural façade,

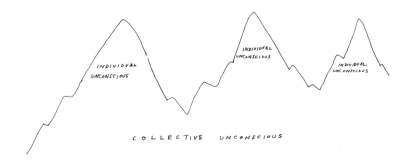

Figure 7.1

as the movement of populations among other things demonstrates, when people from anywhere else integrate with the host culture.

The archetypes formed the contents of the collective unconscious as an inherited archive, and were often described by Jung in terms of folklore images of forms and figures like the hero, the chief, the great mother, the all-merciful, the magician, the monster, and so on. This is where I believe Jung's theory, one of the most important I think in the history of psychology, was driven off the road by people having read only some of what he said, because what came down to us through many popular accounts was that Jung proposed that we inherited actual ideas and imagery; a kind of psychic Lamarckism, as if we could see in our minds' eyes something our ancestors had seen: hence we might 'see' a dragon in a bad dream. Or 'know' what a dragon is like in a children's story, because an ancestor had been chased by a reptile. Jung did refute this, and found he had to reiterate that archetypes were not inherited ideas (or images for that matter) but inherited *possibilities* of ideas. To enlarge on the snapping crocodile on page 104, I don't believe I have inherited an inner picture of a dinosaur, but I am prepared to believe that my mind might have evolved equipped with the wherewithal to be wary if confronted with large, leaping, slavering scaly shapes approaching at speed.

'Archetypes are factors and motives', Jung said, 'which along with instincts arrange elements in the mind so as to form images which may be called archetypal ... they represent psychic instances of the patterns of behaviour which are known to the biologist and which determine the specific manner of all living creatures. Just as the manifestations of this basic biological plan can change in the course of development, so too can the archetypes'. Further, he concluded that these elements were neural (Jung 1954).

However, especially if you can see convincing aspects to archetypal hypotheses, bear in mind that they remain controversial at best and ignored or derided at worst in many mainstream academic circles; this despite recent support for the existence of equivalent mechanisms (though typically not described as archetypal) emerging from linguistics and the most recent neuroscience (*see* p. 106 and Chapter 9).

Archetypes, intuition and the active imagination

I have given archetypal psychology a key place in this account of consciousness because it provides a mechanism for the recognition of people, places and things which one hasn't personally experienced, the simplest though perhaps most important example being a new mother knowing what a baby is, what it is like, what it needs and how it feels to look after it; and, correspondingly, the baby's recognition of a human face. Critics (for example, see Jean Knox, below) would argue *but* the child doesn't, indeed couldn't, have within itself an image of a human face to recall. I would say that this doesn't acknowledge adequately (a) that you don't have to possess an actual picture in the head (indeed the exact neurological nature of an image remains mysterious), and what is important is the brain's capacity to generate imagery from nerve networks within and stimuli from without, thus creating something big, new, affect-laden and vivid (e.g. mother and baby) from scanty-seeming ingredients; and (b) that somewhere in the controversy is a misunderstanding of the nature of memory. Memory isn't 'past' – memory is now. If I recollect, say, images from my childhood (I can just recall a few moments in a pram and the smell or taste of its plastic lining) or episodes at school, indeed many hundreds or even thousands of hours of the past, one has a sense of 'pastness' – many people say it is like looking backwards down a kind of tunnel, accompanied by a strong sense of passing years – yet all that is *right now*, in the head, and nowhere else. 'The War', or whatever else people may recollect, occupies a past existence of sorts which seems very real, especially when reinforced by other people's agreement about what happened and by all the books, films and archives, but there is no past outside the imagination; nor any future. Rather, past and future are like two brilliant pieces of epic cinema, projected back and forth from milliseconds of present brain activity.

To return to the concept of archetypes – a baby recognising a mother's face, let us say – this is not an image recalled from millions of years of successful evolution, but something the baby can do *now* (indeed has yet to do, in the next few moments, if one is thinking of experimental observations) as a new, creative act using what its innate nerve network makes of the outside world. It is a new act of reality-based imagination each time, not something called up from the archives in the basement.

If one talks about intuition, gut feelings about a situation, or even 'ancient wisdom', the temptation is to assume that something psychologically tangible has been drawn up from unknown depths, and that is readily refuted. But what it is more likely to be is creative work of an experienced nervous system a thousand million years in the making in processing present data and coming to a conclusion about what the world is like.

A common example: many people meeting, say, royalty or a 'Big Star' or powerful people, perhaps a personal hero or heroine, often report a strong sense of awe, though the coolest may deny it. You may observe facial expressions and body language demonstrating this in newsreels. But why? Why, for example, did so many people feel such grief on the death of the Princess of Wales? Why was a democratic left-wing Labour MP shown pictured head down, leaning forward earnestly from his chair and looking up in the most submissive and respectful seeming of postures when filmed a couple of years ago meeting Saddam Hussein? Consider the facial expressions in the old newsreels of people meeting Adolf Hitler. I am convinced that what we are seeing in all such situations is what happens when the human psyche meets any sort of cultural icon or iconic situation: there is a sparking both ways, just as lightning strikes rapidly up and down, the man- (and mind-) made icon, the archetype without, recognised and flooded with feelings by the archetype within, accompanied by a barrage of projected feelings and assumptions.

Otherwise, why feel so powerfully about someone you don't know? It could be a figure not at all famous, but representing a group you are prejudiced about in either direction. Would someone feel the same about any figure, prominent or otherwise but fitting an archetypal bill, who turned out to have been played by an actor, even an imposter? Of course, yes. And what is, say, a King or Queen or president but someone playing an archetypal King or Queen or president, and in my view none the worse for that. Back to Genet and his balcony again.

Archetypes, evolution and the self

Anthony Stevens (1982, 1993, 2002), who more than anyone else has explored Jung's original ideas in the light of ethology and evolution, describes archetypes as 'universal forms of instinctive and social behaviour as well as universally recurring symbols and motifs' and which are evolutionary in their development, subserving survival no less than do anatomical and physiological structures and reflex activities (1982). What is particularly interesting in the context of consciousness is Stevens' criticism of ethology (that is, evolutionary behaviourists) in being concerned with overt behaviour rather than with inner, subjective experience (2002). Stevens points out that while ethological studies connect archetypal experience to the outside world of life, behaviour and survival, Jung's psychology made connections with inner awareness. Jung saw the archetypal process as mediating between conscious and unconscious minds and considered it extraordinary that an event which occurs outside produces simultaneously an inner image. Thus it also occurs within; in other words it becomes conscious. He suggested that we are able to be conscious of what we don't know of the world and the cosmos because we are aware of the equivalent division within, which to me is an interestingly quantitative rather than qualitative version of an archetype. Awareness of what is as yet unknown is perhaps a prerequisite of curiosity and exploration.

Jean Knox, in one of the most thorough and wide-ranging recent reviews of the nature of archetypes (2003), distils from many sources four main categories of concept. First, the *genetic* (my headings): sets of instructions for mind and body contained 'hard-wired' within the genes; second, the *developmental*: organising mental frameworks of an abstract nature with no symbolic representational content but which are primitive and are consistent with the period from early psychological development onwards, and which do not have and do not need a genetic basis; third, *emergent brain properties* as the brain interacts with narrative and its environment, as described by Saunders and Skar (2001); and, fourth, *metaphysical entities* which are eternal and independent of the body and representing a transcendental reality, which refers again to Plato's ideal forms (*see* p. 106). These, while seeming at first as if a long way from science, may actually represent rules of mathematics which, I would assume, would apply whatever universe came into being and in that sense would antedate it; and like fractals (*see* p. 63) produce repeated similar patterns in the natural and inanimate world and could similarly determine how the brain categorises information from without and within. (*See* for example McDowell 2001.) Knox (2003) concludes that archetypes are in her third category as emergent brain properties, products of early mental development, capable of further development into the world of imagination and metaphor, and potentially consistent with McDowell's mathematical principles, but that they are not innate, genetic structures. She argues that there cannot be specific archetypes (like a mother figure) because they would require more representational content than is possible; and draws attention to conceptual slippage between archetypes as organising structures and archetypes as conveying (through the genes) core meanings, which she says is 'pure Lamarckism' and with which even Jung would have disagreed.

Jean Knox's critical arguments are important for the development of the archetypal concept. Her argument, though clearly presented, deals with highly complex subjects and I may not have understood crucial points she makes. They leave me with two main questions, however. First, in the light of the way genetics is believed to work I am uncertain what brain processes can be said to be entirely non-genetic. Presumably the way a brain works, whether affected by McDowell's eternal mathematical rules or by the kind of experience a child has during early development, is likely to be influenced by the anatomy, physiology and chemistry with which it is endowed? If someone develops a phobia or a depressive state or for that matter is a significant artist or poet or offender they do not have to have actually inherited any of these conditions or qualities in a way that could be charted out on a genogram; one could postulate a hundred specific traits that could load the dice for the emergence of an artist, a poet, a disorder or a criminal, without any need for an artistic or criminal or illness gene. But the kind of brain it is, its limitations and possibilities, and how it interacts with its own subsequent experience, is still influenced by the genes which made it.

Second, Jean Knox expresses doubt about the possibility of core meaning being inherited, and argues that this represents Lamarckism. I think the problem is how far one is prepared to take the elaboration of the self-organising principle of the brain. If small advantage matters in evolution, tipping the balance just enough for survival and reproduction, I do not see why self-organisation cannot be quite fine tuned, so that the infant with the *potentiality* to form an ever-more detailed image *and* its accompanying feelings (perhaps of love, safety and subjective warmth in nearness) is at an advantage in the attachment lottery compared with a sibling or cousin, say, slightly less well equipped, and as with language, the capacity for new learning during development will be modulated by innate influences too. Thus the developing infant, recognising a 'usable' image of a mother figure in real life as if through archetypal perception, is then in a position to respond and add new learning as it develops. Without that image, learning might not have been able to start.

Thus I do not see the 'mother figure' (or any other archetype) as *ever* needing to be quite as representational as Jean Knox suggests before she argues that it cannot be innate. Regarding the findings that infants do appear to be born with an innate knowledge of the human face (Johnson and Morton 1991) she points out that this important, innate capability need be no more than an orientating response to a particular stimulus, and that psychological representations could emerge through later learning. Both are true, but for me affirm the existence and beauty of the archetypal process which, with reference to the earlier remark about memory and the active imagination, could well include the basic neural circuit board *and* what was then built upon it. Sherrington's 'busy loom of the brain' comes to mind again, and my own conception of an infant's image of a mother figure is of layered part-images, part-memories, part-fantasies and multiple feelings rapidly being scanned by the emerging self while the 'object' in the real world is similarly fast-scanned and compared with the changing inner imagery; something which from moment to moment takes a shape not 'as' a mother figure but enough like a mother figure to serve a transient purpose, before the latter is picked up by further experience, development and learning. Meanwhile, I recommend Jean Knox's important book.

Summary: the birth of an archetype

One must imagine a hypothetical ancestor in new territory, an early ape-like creature, innocent of the danger of a particular predator. Let us say that so far it has innate fight, fright and flight tendencies if anything strange comes along, but does not discriminate so well between various new animals it is discovering, some of whom it will hunt and some of whom will hunt our remote relative.

1   Imaginary creatures are exposed to predator P. (*See* Figure 7.2.)
2   One of the creatures, C, has a variation in its neural system that makes it better able to discriminate aspects of P's shape onto which

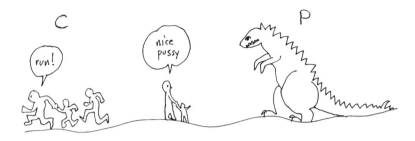

Figure 7.2

it projects inner awareness of danger. Without being aware of how it does it, because of C's 'abnormality' compared with the others it is able to categorise P as potential diner rather than dinner, and flees. Several of the others stay behind, one joining the predator for lunch. (*See* Figure 7.3.)

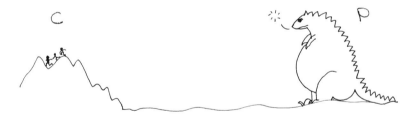

Figure 7.3

3　C survives, and its descendants have neural systems on balance better able to pick up and perceive the shape and meaning of P than its fellows (*see* Figure 7.4), who continue to be eaten.

4　The new C species that populates the area has the internal equivalent of a photographic plate – *not* with an 'image' of P on it but the neural equivalent of a dark room, able to generate in the external world an image of P and attribute dangerous things to it. This was a chance variation, further encouraged in C's descendants by P eating those without the variation. But the experience of C has acted on *species* C, i.e. C's descendants, so that C's fortuitous

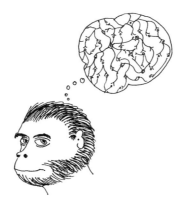

Figure 7.4 ... not an image in the mind, but the innate neural capacity to form an image in the mind ...

sensitivity (or 'paranoia') about P has become perpetuated as a characteristic of those who inherit C's genes.

5 Thus in *genetic*, not developmental terms, the C species now has an imprint recording one of myriad interactions with its environment, which includes not the image of the beast but the *capacity to perceive qualia* and objective characteristics of P – like fast-approaching shapes focused on the observer as they thunder over the ground, or perhaps with flapping, frightening, fast-descending dark shapes dropping from the sky.

Later descendants of C may be able to imagine these kinds of frights, embellish them with what they see around them, and in due course create myths or write books about dragons, which strikes a receptive chord in readers – also descendants of C – even though they don't know why, any more than they know why some of them are repulsed by spiders, and others by snakes. (*See* Figure 7.5.)

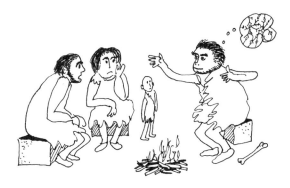

Figure 7.5 Tales told about monsters around the fire (or in the pub)

Conclusion

The idea for an archetypal process that I have described here is not quite the conventional one. It is the hypothesis that a general characteristic of those aspects of the nervous system which form the roots of the mind is that they are economically fine-tuned not only to the material environment but to the emotional climate too; and also to the inward and outward perceptions of the emergent 'I'. If archetypal processes and phenomena are as fundamental to mind and consciousness as a large minority think, it is inherently likely that their source is multifactorial, arising from many genes and the outcome of many genetic–environmental interactions. The idea that archetypes represent a unitary phenomenon seems to me an example of the essentially flawed nature of applying 'either/or' thinking to biological and psychological processes. I prefer the kind of account Lyons (1988) makes in a different (though related) context, the nature and origin of language: that it is 'a multi-layered or multi-stranded phenomenon, each of whose layers or strands may be of different antiquity and different origin'. I believe this is the only way to think of mental development and phenomena, however inconvenient.

Meanwhile, it seems to me that archetypes as described by Jung, indeed by Plato, and as reviewed in Jean Knox's critical account, represent particular and comparatively circumscribed examples of what is actually a wider general characteristic of our innate neural repertoire.

8

What the poets know

Art: the artist as visionary, magician, explorer and clown

> It is not that the artist is a special kind of man. Man is a special kind of artist.
>
> *(AK Cooramaswamy 1950)*

Arts

I have invoked arts and artistry throughout this book, and in this chapter want to draw a few threads together. In casting about for a definition of art that would get away from framed art and gallery or concert-hall art, I appreciated the Oxford English Dictionary for defining art as 'skill, human skill as opposed to nature ... thing in which skill may be exercised'. This is what I mean by art, consistent with my quote from Cooramaswamy.

I don't exclude 'big art' by recognised artists of every kind, from painting to poetry and music to film-making, and I have tended to refer to known names as well as unknown artists – and apes. However, rather than place all human artistry as if in a minor echelon compared with seriously recognised art, I would reverse their respective positions, and suggest that for the study of art's role in consciousness all human musings, scribblings and scratchings from the most trivial through the mediocre, banal and unrecognised to the competent is what matters, compared with which classical art represents a bonus.

If you were to ask a hundred people at random where they would rate art in importance in everyday life, I suspect art and artists would rank pretty low compared with, say, brain surgeons and engineers; if one threw in poets too, that would really lower art's score. Yet the visiting alien whose judgement we often value would be astonished at the artistic output of planet earth: even in a silent room the airwaves are packed with wall-to-wall music and lyrics in hundreds if not thousands of broadcasts, round the clock, as turning on and tuning a radio receiver would show. Add to this design and illustration everywhere – pictures, papers, cards, wallpaper, clothes, fashion, cars, houses, architecture, and add cooking, photography, sports, cinema, television ... we wade through this constant outpouring of creativity, good, bad and indifferent, as though through a flood in torrential rain, yet still think of 'art' as something a little peculiar and somewhat sidelined. Meanwhile, the most prominent and highly paid people by far, our 'stars' and gods, are artists or 'artistes' of one sort or another. We are immersed in art, as suspended in art as Bohr said (1963) we are suspended in language. To such forms of art I would add craftsmanship too; as David Pye (1968) says in his classic account of the nature and art of workmanship, there is a balance to be achieved between precision and approximation, regulation and freedom, every formal element having a maximum and a minimum effective range, and the product of good workmanship has its own aesthetic and style and is good for us. All this is very close to the idea of teeming memes too (*see* p. 70) in terms of output if not necessarily in terms of the concept of replication and selection.

Art and consciousness

The model for consciousness I am proposing is circular. I don't believe animals think about what they make, although the bird in its nest or the rabbit in its burrow will have some inner representation and awareness of its home on its general territorial map. I have argued that humans, however, rather like track-laying vehicles, throw out things generated from themselves upon which to advance their exploration and their thinking; the metaphor I used earlier as the grappling hook: a projection, perhaps an idea or a phrase, sent out as a feeler; for example, to see if a menacing-seeming situation is actually danger-ous, or whether a sound sent out produces a response in the hearer. And, whatever the reaction, the result comes back like the signal of an echo-sounder, not only telling us where we are and with whom but who we are. Do appreciate that I am thinking metaphors here – not only the actual physical feedback, though that is just as important. In this sense we constantly stitch ourselves into the external world, surrounding ourselves with a complexly woven nest of familiar people, places, things, ideas and artefacts, and particularly ideas and artefacts. In this way we furnish our lives, and, I would argue, our conscious-ness. If you can empty your mind of all of this, you might find little left, indeed be in a much sought-after meditative state of mindlessness; or fall asleep. More likely, it may be quite difficult to leave the mental world of thoughts, images and objects behind.

There is also the art of other people. We speak, and people speak back in symbolic sounds that convey feeling and meaning. The echoes we receive back through our echo-sounder contain so much that is recognised as familiar that the unfamiliar is readily recognised too; which is where I would place the archetypes discussed in Chapter 7. This potential-for-imagery forged from a negotiation between our surging unconscious, animal selves and the *socio-cultural* aspects of evolution can become actual inner, affect-laden images once the potential-for-imagery is projected onto the 'canvas' outside. For example, someone proposes a quite new person to meet, place to go or thing to do, and immediately we project imagery, stereotypes, prejudgements, to start turning over the engines of anticipation and preparedness, the vivid imagery for which is generated from the dull blueprints of the archetypes in the neural network.

The point about archetypes is that they are shared. A stereotype can be quite superficial, personal, idiosyncratic and possibly quickly dispelled by whatever the reality turns out to be. Archetypes are more rooted and enduring, and are shared not just because they occupy the collective unconscious but are behind whole swathes of our visible, audible, tangible culture, out there in an elaborate, kaleidoscopically changing pattern of sounds, words, signs, symbols and images, designed and made by people with minds like ours for minds like ours, on signposts, in the way buildings, towns and cities are designed and places shaped and landscaped, in books and shop windows and on billboards, stage and screen. One way or another, they help make up our minds.

This is what I mean by the mind making the culture and the culture making the mind, and to the extent that managing relationships is an art I would include much of the findings and theory of anthropology within my formula of mind generates art and art feeds mind. But for this chapter I will confine myself to the more materially 'made' arts.

Art, expression, culture

Among her many illuminating accounts of the philosophy and psychology of art, Susanne Langer (1953) wrote, with reference to music, but also to art in general, that expression is a state of mind yet represents other things too – customs, dress, behaviour 'and [reflects] confusion or decorum, violence or peace'. And humour too, I would add: how can phrases of music seem witty, even hilarious? Doesn't the Laurel and Hardy signature tune ('Waltz of the Cuckoos') *sound* like how an incongruous procession of two people heading with vulnerable dignity towards a fall might look or feel? Is that because we mentally enact or imagine physical movements to the music that, if we were to perform them, would make us feel like that and laugh; just as martial music produces the feel or fantasy of marching. Thus the James-Lange hypothesis – another 'reversal' model – that physiological changes can result in a relevant emotion, rather than the other way round. This, I think, is where art and consciousness merge – the mix comes from, yet feeds and informs, not just culture and physiology but our joints and movements, our very appearance and purposes. Langer (1953) goes further: the tonality of music also conveys:

> *growth and attenuation, flowing and stowing, conflict and resolution, speed, arrest, terrific excitement, calm, or subtle activation and dreamy lapses ... such is the pattern, or logical form, of sentience; and the pattern of music is that same form worked out in pure, measured sound and silence. (Langer 1953)*

And isn't this, the sound, the balance, the muscles, nerves and joints, the dress too, an account of dance? But besides all these, Langer continues, the art will also express 'the unconscious wishes and nightmares of its author'. I hope that thought is just a little alarming.

But this is all, as it were, what we know, or can know. What about being in the dark about art? Referring to the sculpture of Henry Moore and his view that making art is a primordial experience, Read (1960) is with Jung (1922) that the artist is somehow outside, even beneath, his or her art, is a kind of conduit who doesn't know where the art comes from or is leading to. On the one hand this may be an interesting comment on art. I think it is also a remarkable comment on consciousness; or, to bring things down to earth a little, on the brain, on people. Read also refers to aesthetic imagery as reconciling, in relation to the conflict between, for example, spirit and instinct, the uncivilised (or pre-cultural) and the civilised, or self with the 'absurdity of existence'.

The tragi-comedy inherent in this use of the word absurdity may remind us of the importance in culture of the art of the clown, comedian, and fool, the latter being the historical word for jester, as in the Court Jester who was allowed, indeed wanted, to fill the ambiguous role of subservience to the ruler whom he also mocked.

This paradoxically affirmed the ruler's authority while challenging it. We see the same when a comic interviewer jokes about the celebrity guest; it invites the assumption that this must be a great man or woman indeed (perhaps greater even than was thought) to be impervious to such impertinence. But at another level, the everyday one, the tease, with its nice mixture of empathy and sadism, is an ambiguous invitation to the ordinary self to stand up for itself, to be intact enough to stand outside itself, see its vulnerability in relation to its much greater strengths, and share in the humour. Small wonder that some troubled people – children with autistic spectrum disorders, for example, distressed by the emotional arousal and cognitive ambiguity of teasing – can find being teased devastating. The experience is a sharpened, intrusive form of the everyday experience in their development of not knowing how to make something of the ambiguities of life and relationships.

We see the ultimate cultural tease in surrealism, whose project was primarily about floating a whole new psychology that would bring about changes in attitudes and beliefs – or consciousness – by changing the culture. The surrealists thought humanity would be more authentically itself if the gap the surrealists perceived between objectivity and subjectivity, in fact between fantasy and reality, was blurred or better still eliminated. Their work too, which included prose, poetry, writings and dance, while challenging and provocative, also fitted Read's category of reconciling imagery for their public, indeed anyone's public, to make something new with. The surrealists, notably André Breton, were interested in automatism, free association and psychoanalysis, all of which were thought to help in the business of mining the unconscious mind, which, they argued, was best unfettered rather than confined by convention (Breton 1969; Polizzotti 1995; Brandon 1999).

Writing in the 1950s Read identified 'certain works of contemporary art' as constituting such imagery and considered it unprecedented. He chose Kandinsky, Picasso (perhaps the first surrealist painter with his 1925 *Three Dancers*), Mondrian, Gabo and Moore. 'All these artists have in common a will to create images that are metaphysical, beyond the limits of the phenomenal world.' However, with this compliment came the warning that 'no number of unscrupulous imitators can take away the significance' of these new plastic images (Read, 1960). But, half a century later, can we tell the difference between the real thing and the imitator? And would not the dyed-in-the-wool surrealist – and their successors – revel in the idea of the challenge of the genuinely bogus? If *anything* can be art, even non-art or anti-art, and if its purpose is to make us think, to provoke and to shock, where does that leave art? As a kind of spiritual-political movement? Perhaps so, with the most provocative, the headline-makers, either as fundamentalists or fools. Cecil Collins, visionary artist, identified the Fool as embodying saint, artist and poet, who stands for a 'purity of consciousness' – a kind of transparent honesty, I think – whose 'purity is cosmic folly that is utterly detached from what the world thinks worth doing ... the Fool must not exist in men, for the Fool is interested in life, not in power, nor in the accumulation of knowledge, nor in the passing of examinations, nor in being clever' (Collins 1989; Keeble 1994). He was not impressed by the surrealists, seeing them as inventing reality, and as materialists, or at least dialectical materialists, valuing matter over thought. The task of the Fool, Collins argued, was engagement with spiritual reality. The free-floating fantasies of surrealism came from inchoate regions which did not enable cognition to engage with the real, and allowed consciousness no context.

Comparing surrealism with Collins' visionary art, which has been compared to that of William Blake's in importance, I think Collins' prospectus is the more revolutionary. But surrealism was not the end of its particular line, and should no more be rejected than psychoanalysis, whose detractors, as with surrealism, tend to focus on (or only be aware of) fragments of both, and of their *forme frustes*. Thus Leja (1993) describes American Abstract Expressionists of the 1940s like Jackson Pollock, Mark Rothko and Willem de Kooning as continuing in the United States where the surrealism of Europe left off, or as some would say got into a dead end. Leja sees their work as 'part of a culture-wide initiative to re-imagine the Self', their understanding inspired by Freudian and Jungian thinking, and aligns them with many writers and film-makers of the period. (And see Fineberg 2000.)

What about the many people who privately paint or draw or write poetry or fiction for their own need or interest, with no particular intention of ever showing the work to, let alone influencing, anybody? There are also 'outsider' artists, self-taught painters, sculptors and others who work just for themselves, some of whom are psychologically unwell or eccentric or socially isolated, and if in a sense they are speaking to themselves through their art, perhaps this represents a short-circuit in my (now-mixed) metaphor of 'throwing the grappling iron'; here, mind may be speaking to self for personal clarification or relief, rather than for communication. Yet 'outsider' art has also become blurred at the edges with folk art, which by definition is embedded in a community. There is art that reinforces the sense of self, art for informing others' selves, and the 'delayed action' information of self and others that is routed through the culture. There are such haunting resonances between the work of such artists who have never met others or seen each other's work that it does indeed give the impression of raw art from the depths, practically primary art straight from the brain and the soul, and possibly tells us something about the creative, disturbing and perhaps disturbed roots of humanity (see Thevoz 1976; Cardinal 1972; Prinzhorn 1995; Williams 1992; Maizels 1996; Brand-Claussen *et al.* 1997), particularly in the context of Stevens', Price's and Horrobin's ideas about human origins discussed below (*see* pp. 128,129).

Art, science, spirituality

We can be touched to unknown depths by corresponding unknown depths in art, music, prose and poetry: we all have different ways of describing physiological experiences – e.g. goose pimples – caused by immaterial abstractions. Emily Dickinson, quoted by Camille Paglia (2001), said 'if I read a book and it makes my whole body feel that no fire can ever warm me I know *that* is poetry. If I feel physically as if the top of my head were taken off, I know *that* is poetry'. Paglia herself says 'poetry is assault and battery on the body'. In her book Paglia relates physical sexuality and gender to poetry and the certain passion and violence there, exemplified in Dickinson's work. Is that something spiritual arising from and to an extent beyond the animal and material? Frank Avray Wilson (1958, 1963, 1981), abstract painter, biologist and philosopher, has referred to the essential 'otherness' of art, and how it has been provoked by the challenge from nature 'as generous mother, lover, persecutor or tormentor' (Wilson, 1958), to which I would add these as fantasies as well as material realities; and Wilson (1981) refers to abstract art as an assertive, almost aggressive effort in the interests of personal existence to reach and express another, less material, more magical world, and which he sees as transcendental. God has been described as 'God of the (as yet) unknown' and similarly perhaps spirituality is what seems to be still there and unaccounted for when we have described as best we can the Self. The 'otherness' of art, its essential abstraction whatever its material forms, is why I think it is properly associated with the non-natural, and in this may come close to being in a not natural yet non-supernatural category of existence, along with spirituality, something discussed further in Chapter 11.

But what *is* the spiritual? Do we need it? If we have instincts, intelligence and feelings, and accept unconscious as well as conscious processes in the mind, is there a place for the spiritual? Jung (1928) associated it with the archetypes, but one that arose *sui generis*, and with the instincts, but saw it as in conflict with what he called blind instinctivity. Here we have a conceptual problem, especially with Jaques Maritain's case (1954) for the illuminating intellect which is spiritual but *does not know*, presumably in the cognitive sense, but only activates. Aristotle said nothing could be found in the intellect which didn't come *via* the senses as fantasies and images of material things. Maritain, theologian and aesthetic philosopher, suggests that it is more complicated than this, and in a statement which is certainly complex but also I think is precise describes the intelligible content in images as only potentially intelligible 'or capable *of being made capable*' of becoming an object of intellectual vision. This is what the un-knowing but activating illuminating intellect does: 'impregnating the intellect' by the 'impressed pattern or intelligible germ' and resulting in the spiritual. It is a convoluted argument, but to me is consistent with a process by which archetypes produce 'I' from the dawning intellect and in turn *shape* the developing intellect in a process that spirals – that is, moves further with every turn of the cycle – towards something quite new, which might be within oneself or outside on a sheet of music or on a canvas, yet which is ultimately powered from something 'old' in the sense of always there – timeless. In his essay *On the Spiritual in Art*, Kandinsky (1946) makes the point that all these (created) forms, when truly artistic, become food for the spirit. Does 'spirituality', whether acknowledged or not, enable and power curiosity about *what else* there could be and where and how to find it?

The process is, in a way, a drawing from the depths to make something 'in here' or 'out there' which then nourishes, sustains and informs the depths, and I would link the idea with archetypal activity and common to art and spirituality, both of which represent something within the mind but also *beyond the mind*, which seems to be echoed in the cosmologist John Barrow's argument for 'unexpected ways in which the structure of the Universe – its laws, its environments and its astronomical appearance – imprints itself upon our thoughts, our aesthetic preferences, and our views about the nature of things' (Barrow 1995) and with the notion of the anthropic principle

(Davies 1982; Barrow and Tipler 1986; Davies and Brown 1986) which reminds us that in a quantum physics understanding of the universe (observable in action in experiments) the 'observer' is actually part of the performance and that – if I am accurately condensing a complicated hypothesis – our understanding of the universe, everything from our aesthetic and poetic representation of the universe, conceivably even such ineffable phenomena as intuition and synchronicity, all the way to the scientific laws we 'discover' about the universe, *fit* the universe because our minds are shaped by these same laws (*see* p. 96). We make the universe as the universe makes us.

Networks within and without

Although the grappling hook model is partly about reality testing, communicating and connecting, it also operates within, reflecting from self back to self. Writers and other artists know the experience of having ideas in the head which seem clear enough until an attempt is made to make them reasonably precise on the paper or the canvas or on the keyboard – and then the hard work really starts. I would identify three levels, or orbits, in this process: communication to and for oneself; direct communication to others; and communication over time and space. If you crawl into the kind of decorated underground tombs found all over Europe it is difficult not to feel something of what – one imagines – the stone-age stone carvers had in mind, cut and shaped by someone of flesh and blood and no doubt as baffled by it all as we might be ourselves; but human communication at some level is there, likely in this setting to do with existence, perhaps about affirming something lasting despite death, perhaps sharing imagery, perhaps trying to 'fix' in something solid a picture in the artist's head. Perhaps even fulfilment of an inchoate but spiritual feeling of obligation.

To the extent that this happens, and that the projected line is a valid metaphor for what is in effect one of the constant succession of creative experiments with which we find our way around in our worlds, when it actually hooks on and works it provides a basis for others to follow. The successfully thrown lines accumulate as, first, the equivalent of scrambling nets and then as a complex weave connecting self with self and self with other selves. It is a relatively coarse metaphor, but I hope a helpful one; in the abstract, it is about mutuality: mutual understanding, mutual appreciation and shared culture. In Chapter 9 I will be looking at the matrix within the head – the neural network – that underwrites the physical components of consciousness. This elaborate network of reality testing, mutuality, shared ideas and conceptions and relationships, and the representation of these abstractions in material form – art, drama, architecture, activities – represents a cultural mirroring without of the neural network within. Imagery straddles both: the imagery within one self, the imagery in other selves, and the making of material imagery in the solid, external world.

David Lewis-Williams (2002), interestingly reversing the issue in his book's subtitle *consciousness and the origin of art*, suggested that cave-paintings were an attempt by palaeolithic man to deal with emerging consciousness, which he properly distinguishes from intelligence alone. They needed to do something with their mental imagery, in which Lewis-Williams supposed hallucinations formed a part, and to fix them – metaphorically as well as literally – onto cave walls, perceiving these boundaries to their safest areas as 'the membrane between their world and the spirit world from which they came'. Whether anyone could know whether they experienced what we would technically identify as true hallucinations (as opposed to vivid internal imagery, illusions or fantasies), I think it is reasonable to suppose that emotive imagery is likely to lead to the attempt to make sense of it to oneself and others and to set it down for reflection, recollection and communication. To the extent that it was potent stuff from the spirit world it could be better also to 'earth it', spirits being not necessarily all-powerful but beings one could deal with one way or another. The imagery was better out than in, perhaps, and none the less important for that. Some have suggested that elaborately decorated caves may represent the earliest forms of what became cathedrals, although Bahn (2005) has disputed that they necessarily represented early centres for religious activity, since the inaccessibility of some notable examples made it seem that they were designed to remain *hidden*; though for me this sounds particularly like their having a proto-religious purpose.

Art and curiosity

If art represents a reaching beyond the known (and perhaps unwelcome or intolerable) to something else, to another kind of explanation, one that others might appreciate too, it would have some of the characteristics of spirituality and meet an important evolutionary requirement too – for human curiosity, without which, as I argued earlier, we would never had been motivated to use brains or muscle. The sense of conviction that goes with art – the authority of the author too, which makes printed marks come alive in the reader's mind – is also importance in adaptation. Absolute belief in oneself or an enterprise may lead to catastrophe or success (Wolpert, 2006), but nature isn't upset by many failures if a few successes get through, and the human capacity for *conviction* has evolutionary advantage.

More often art, and I think spirituality too, regularly function as repositories of incomplete ideas, attitudes and feelings until one makes up one's mind about them, or even if one never does. Another adaptive human characteristic in human evolution and in mature people is the capacity to live with uncertainty and ambiguity; it is to wonder without knowing, to be curious without any evidence that curiosity will be satisfied, soon or ever. This, to me, is not only like art, where one can discern enough meaning or find enough enjoyment without being quite sure why, perhaps not for years, but also rather like what in psychoanalytic theory and practice are known as transitional objects, holding the situation or idea while, consciously or unconsciously, work is done on it. I have read poetry and books or seen films or heard music that I didn't like much at the time, yet have hung around on the fringes of consciousness until, much later, I have revisited them, and found them not merely alight but – occasionally – enormously rewarding. Winnicott (1972) identified transitional objects as occupying an intermediate place between the imagination (and of course the fears, fantasies, wishes and assumptions of the imagination) and reality, and identified this position as cultural. It can be conceived as a tentative and transitory container for consciousness, or a kind of holding zone while minds are made up.

Winnicott recognised the tentativeness and ambivalence in this intermediate position when he wrote:

> In the artist of all kinds I think one can detect an inherent dilemma, which belongs to the co-existence of two trends, the urgent need to communicate and the still more urgent need not to be found. This might account for the fact that we cannot conceive of an artist's coming to the end of the task that occupies his whole nature.

On the one hand this may seem the vaguest of prospectuses; and yet it is very close to the most enduring and productive philosophy of science – specifically that of Karl Popper (Miller 1983; Popper

1999), where all facts are necessarily provisional, leading primarily to further curiosity, more questions, more refutations of hypotheses and then the emergence of provisional facts and working, practical, but still provisional knowledge.

Earlier (p. 58) I related 'making sense' to paranoia – making up one's mind on inadequate evidence. This is surely a continuous and compelling thread in human history. Spirituality, art, myths, fantasy and dreams are all ways of holding situations, thinking about them after a fashion, even coming to part-solutions and provisional, working conclusions about things that interest us, and often what they hold for us is as much hope as fear. The anthropologist Joseph Campbell said of dreams 'they are private myths; and myths are public dreams' (Campbell 1974).

The artist as explorer and leader

In earlier chapters I suggested that however much we may value competent action it would need to be preceded by curiosity, motivation and then a degree of hope, recklessness, and gambling; Goethe's wonderful advice 'Whatever you may dream, or think you can, begin it/Boldness has genius, magic and power in it' (Goethe 1832) would have been invaluable for a starving prehistoric family on the wrong side of a river, contemplating a primitive boat. The kind of man or woman I mean might have been a visionary, magician, explorer, clown, artist or some other kind of dramatic innovator, and they and their enterprises would have been subject to rigorous and sometimes brutal natural and unnatural selection. *Following* the artist takes courage too, and often foolhardiness, with practical and social experiments which go disastrously wrong. Prehistorically and historically, these are surely in the vast majority; but that which works (as in evolution) is what we celebrate, whether it is the giraffe's neck or a historic 'success'. Anthony Stevens and John Price have discussed the idea of the charismatic figure, 'disturbed' by modern clinical standards who in particular circumstances might have polarised and split groups and tribes, adopted forms of expression and symbolism that demarcated the 'in-group' from the non-believing enemy, and led their followers off to success, i.e. survival (Stevens and Price 1996). Such adaptive advantage in what they described as a schizophrenic-like condition, its polygenic and multifactorial causation and the apparent relationship between schizophrenia and creativity being associated within the same extended families (as in bipolar disorder too) may explain why it still afflicts 1 person in 100 throughout the world. It is also a reminder how what is a clinical condition in one culture may conceivably have some value in very different circumstance, as was discussed with autistic spectrum disorder (*see* p. 86). David Horrobin's argument that evolutionary developments underlying what we now call schizophrenia caused the emerging human race's complexity, creativity and diversity in thinking and behaviour (Horrobin 2001) is I think consistent with these propositions and also with my own notion of the new primate brain being both an advance and a potential liability. The enormous increase in synaptic complexity accompanying the growth of the to-be-human brain could have raised the curtain on a whole new mental realm of intense cogitating, sometimes wayward and sometimes creative, and whole depths of feelings, fears and fantasies which were quite new for primates yet familiar to ourselves as human beings. I find such theories plausible, especially if we think in terms of gradual changes loading the dice and gradually shaping up how A raises the chances of B happening (e.g. even thinking of crossing the river or splitting with the rest of the group) which influences C and D and so on down the millennia. Gladwell's more general thesis (2002) on how small things can make a big difference and become cultural phenomena is worth reading.

Down the generations there might have been much story-telling about the incident that saved the group that took to the water, doubtless embellished into improving myths, mind speaking to mind down the intervening ages. Need a myth be 'true'? Myth-making is an art, and as the film director Federico Fellini said (1987), when challenged about the factual content of his tales, 'a man is at his most direct and straightforward when he is telling lies. It is when he is trying to tell the truth that he is at his most obscure'.

True, untrue or half-true, the tales told by artists and others (I would include the quantum physicists I have quoted here) represent modern attempts to grasp and explain things which, curiously, seem at once both at the outer edge of the known universe *and* at the outer edge of our consciousness and capacity for understanding. Why does it seem that these apparently quite different things seem to be in the same place? Perhaps there is a clue in the anthropic principle.

Words, language, poetry, evolution

One of the most enchanting suggestions I came across in a long time was the idea that birdsong may have had something to do with the way humans acquired language (Aitchison 1989, 1996). It seems a surprising notion at first, but if one tries to imagine the scene outside the cave, birdsong must surely have stood out remarkably among the roaring, squeaking, grunting and rustling noises and general banging about in the forest and in the cave.

Or, to adopt my own model for how the environmental can become innate, *some* kinds of minds were physically able to appreciate it more than others, and *if* that facilitated language skills and the social skills that flowed from language skills, then those kinds of minds would have had an advantage in achieving predominance.

Social stability is literally vital for social animals. This is not the same as social rigidity. The art here is the art of politics and diplomacy, because, in families, tribes, nations and for that matter in the board-room, there is a time for conservation and a time for revolutionary change. Aitchison (1996) describes two key kinds of behaviour, one to do with maintenance of the pecking order, by which social rank is maintained, and which involves mutual grooming; and the other in which one individual guesses at another's mental state. Anticipating others' minds is a social skill akin to the ability to tell the future, and probably the only reliable form of prophecy in human affairs. Empathy, feeling as if in someone else's place, has its good side in altruism (one of the supposed mysteries of evolution – what on earth is the advantage of selflessness? – so the question goes), but has its other side (what Jung would have called its shadow side) in opening up all sorts of possibilities for deception and deviousness, prominent skills in the great apes, with chimpanzees excelling at it, although human beings are the best.

Aitchison speculates that in an environment where cunning and deviousness were advantageous a large brain would be at an advantage, and she suggests that a large brain could be used to enable the development of 'a superb manipulative device: language' (Aitchison, 1996).

The other side of social stability is the group's ability to change the hierarchy if that is useful and, while this could be achieved, up to a point, by fighting and bloodshed, evolutionary psychiatrists and psychologists (Price 1967; Price and Sloman 1987; Gilbert 1992; Stevens and Price 1996) have suggested another survival-enhancing process by which adolescent apes routinely challenge the dominant ape for the best role, space, wives, food etc. which the dominant ape sees off (not by violence but by the more civilised process of issuing menacing social signals) *until he is no longer up to it*. He then withdraws, becomes less aspirational, and shows many bits of behaviour we would associate with human depression (also associated with actual or symbolic loss of status) except that as human beings we have the consciousness and the language to conceptualise, worry about and express 'depression'. In another part of the jungle, as we saw earlier, Parkes (1969, 1971) has shown how the actual behaviour of animals that have lost a child (agitated, searching behaviour and apparent heightened susceptibility to environmental cues that they may be nearby) is remarkably close to the symptoms of human grief and to how psychoanalysts with no particular knowledge of animal behaviour or ethology have rather poetically described depression and grief: in terms of the 'loss of a loved object'. Apart from their intrinsic interest, these examples also suggest how language and consciousness, if grafted onto essentially primitive, evolved, behaviour patterns, may enable a leap to be made from reflexive behaviour to deeply felt experiences, around which imagery, language, self-awareness and more elaborate, cultural patterns of behaviour can be built. In Chapter 9, we will see how words and language can form a poetry that not only helps shape self and our relationships with the world, but plays a part in the dynamics of attachment and individual development.

Consciousness, place, landscape

Although I have focused on events and relationships, it would be a mistake to exclude place and landscape (Berleant, 2004). These are both powerfully emotive and significant for evolution, in considering the arts of how to live and the archetypes that may become literally incorporated in the species as a result. In exploring the essentials of consciousness, I do not think we should take it for granted that we know how to 'be' up a tree without evolving ways of knowing which way is up, getting up and staying up until we want to come down. Much of the spadework has been done by our animal ancestors, of course. It has been suggested that that sudden feeling of falling and jerking awake, if falling asleep sitting up, was inherited from our time in the trees – possibly with a baby hanging on, or with a predator below. This is not a 'memory of falling', as it is sometimes loosely called; it is an evolved brain capacity. Those without it stood less chance of having descendants. My point is that I don't think we should just take it for granted that a creature of any sort should instinctively assess where it is, where it wants to be and make its way there and stay there for some purpose. After all, a tree or an armchair can't do such things. To take such abilities as simply 'there' is I think to by-pass the foundations of our minds and nervous systems. This is why we sought an evolutionary reason for the single-celled protozoan to move about, to ingest and to excrete.

In keeping with the idea of the founding archetype which *develops* from evolution in the species, and then *guides* perception and learning in each member of that species, I would not assume it was obvious why a creature set down in, say, a new landscape would, without the necessary hard-wiring of the archetype, 'naturally' know what to make of it or what to do with it. Why should it? The creature's nature evolves and learns, and its whole nature develops; thus making something of territory and space – and such things as being interested, being curious, being cautious, exploring, looking and finding, and staying or leaving seem every bit as likely to be rooted in innate capacities as these same characteristics if the creature were observing another beast which might represent food, a prey or danger. That is how deep and detailed I believe we should go in comprehending the evolved particulars of consciousness. An animal *will* assess, instinctively and by learning, the shape, colouring, position, posture, scent and everything else about another living thing relevant to safety or danger, about what to do with it or about it. The emerging, adapting consciousness will do the same with seas, skies, rock, caves, heights, plains and woods and these hard-wired capacities for perception and the *feelings* accompanying these perceptions lay the foundations not just for security and exploration but for a sense of the aesthetics of place. Orians and Heerwagen (1992) in an essay on evolutionary approaches to environmental aesthetics discuss this theme in terms of an imaginary group of adults and children coming across the savannah and the details (characteristically represented in many landscape paintings) which identify what sort of place it is, and what sort of environment it could be for them. It is argued that savannah-type territory was right at the time for early human groups, and recent research demonstrates an aesthetic preference for this type of territory – especially in children under eight years – although from age 15-plus the experience of other types of living space begins to play down the presumed innate preference for savannah. Hepburn (2004) argues that philosophy has underestimated the relationship between the human sense of existence in territory and the aesthetics of landscape.

With our bigger brains and curious capacity for memory and for language, which McCrone (1990) said made all the difference in our evolutionary route from jellyfish to man in terms of the evolving of a sense of self (enabling 'watching the watcher', to which we will return in the next chapter), I suggest we also evolved a far fuller sense of appreciation, beyond simply 'sniffing the air' and beyond necessity, though it now represents a higher appreciativeness which we now take for granted as aesthetics. In his work on films entitled *Kinesics and Context*, Birdwhistell (1970), discussing what seems 'natural' or 'predictable', and imagining the details of reception and transmission in terms of the bits of information about light, sound and odour required for gut feeling, thought that some 2500 to 10 000 bits per second would be needed for the task, a vast number but relatively modest compared with the billion-fold, multi-tasking, attention-switching and focusing capacity of the brain. This represents the undercurrents when, say, a cat enters new territory – albeit quite possibly in a cascade in which large volumes of information quickly cancel each other out and become redundant – and a conclusion about how to respond is reached. As in the cat, so in the classic dramatic situation where people enter what may, or may not, be a menacing old house.

Place and time

John Fowles (1984), writing about Thomas Hardy and Wessex, described novelists as in a sense undertakers, 'concerned to give the past a decent, or at least a thorough, burial'. Isn't this what we all do, one way or another, when making sense of memory when we are not preoccupied with making sense of *now*? In this respect the human race – our writers, historical interpreters, obituarists, reporters, journalists, yarn-spinners and gossips – is like a frantically busy antheap, working round the clock to process what has happened; not, I think, simply for anything so mundane as to affirm or twist aspects of history (after all, there are many exhumations and reburyings of this and that) but as a kind of existential back-up for us, something to be perpetually starting out from.

As novelist and poet – perhaps at his greatest as a poet – Hardy is best known for his writings about places and the way life was lived in a rather small area of Dorset – his 'theatre', as he called it – but even more (or, at least, in a way complementary to this) he was concerned about the passage of time, death, and a melancholy sense of loss. Might his witnessing as a child the execution of Martha Brown (Thorne 2000) outside Dorchester prison have set this off in him? He would still speak mournfully about it years later; and said of life 'that it was a series of fallings from us, vanishings' (Southerington 1971; and James Gibson, personal communication, 2001; see also Hardy, 2000).

Hardy was a psychologist before the profession was created. It is not surprising that in his last novel *The Well-Beloved* (1897) he anticipated Jung's archetypal psychology by half a century; as we have seen such ideas were in the air, that is to say in our consciousness, since Plato. In this book, one that at least one critic thought should have been burned, the protagonist falls in love successively with a woman, her daughter and her grand-daughter, seeing in each an ideal image of the woman he wants, something he makes more explicit in his poem of the same name. When striding across the Island of Portland *en route* to see the 'real' person, a spirit falls into step beside him and asserts that it is *she* – though unattainable – that he really wants. Now, this is not by any means a unique theme in fiction, nor in life, but here the artist produces it out of a hat – or out of his head – as something at a level that lies between mere psychology and ordinary narrative, uniting yet dividing both. Hardy kept notes on the emerging proto-psychology of the day, and one of his biographers, Rosemary Sumner, described *The Well-Beloved* as largely a vehicle for his ideas, which spanned the psychological and the biological (Bullen 1994), saying that 'there is underlying all the fantasy followed by the visionary artist the truth that all men are pursuing a shadow, the unattainable' (Sumner 1981). And he also said (Sumner 1981) 'if you mean to make the world listen, you must say what they will all be thinking and saying five and twenty years hence'. Thus, the grappling hook again, the long-flung version, and one that takes hold. It is neither just predictive, nor creative, but both.

Robert Smithson, who designed the extraordinary *Spiral Jetty* which extends a quarter of a mile into the Great Salt Lake, Utah, was on the face of it an artist in earth, rocks and landscape, but his understanding of the way concepts of territory and time were fused was as natural as any geologist's. In his essay 'Entropy and the new monuments' (1979) he discusses the Monumental – huge, enduring public works from work like his own to New York apartment buildings as capturing place, space and time, though encapsulating time's paradox too, that we lose it as we gain it. *Spiral Jetty*, built in the 1970s in what were thought to be static waters, disappeared beneath the surface of its lake in the 1980s, but by the later 1990s has been slowly coming to the surface again. No doubt it will rise and fall, marking the passage of time and geography. Smithson was killed in an air crash in 1973 while surveying another project. Gary Shapiro provides an account of the work and thought of this extraordinary time traveller, with the roots of his ideas in the philosophy of Hegel, and Hegel's identification of the Tower of Babel with the monumental, necessarily public work of art whose purpose is meant to focus a general attention on whatever it is that is vital to the way a community understands itself (Shapiro 1995). Such works of art, artefact and myth are cultural versions of the carbon clock. They help fix ourselves in time and space, a vital, consciousness-sustaining network of things and ideas. In his essay *The Shape of Time* George Kübler makes an equivalent point about less monumental things – 'the whole range of man-made things, including all tools and writing in addition to the useless, beautiful and poetic things of the world. By this view the universe of man-made things simply coincides with the history of art' (Kübler 1962) – and, I would say, the history and development of consciousness. 'Such things', Kübler argues, 'mark the passage of time with far greater accuracy than we can know ... like crustaceans we depend for survival upon an outer skeleton, upon a shell of historic cities and houses filled with things belonging to definable portions of the past.' The French philosopher Bachelard in *The Poetics of Space* (1964) made a similar point in relation to such physical and mental furniture as 'shells and door-knobs, closets and attics, old towers and peasant huts', providing containers for metaphor, imagination and humanness (Stilgoe, in his Foreword, 1964).

Malraux (1958) described the cinema as an industry which aimed to set the whole world dreaming, and defined the moment when it moved from recording scenes to true expression when directors began to experiment with space, time and camera position, all in a sequence of planes. The Russian director Andrey Tarkovsky identified film and photography as uniquely concerned with time. In his book *Sculpting in Time* (1986) he related the cinematic and photographic with memory and with *knowing*, which he 'dates' mythically from Eve eating the apple from the tree of knowledge, and in historical terms as a never-ending task, because it represents a yearning for an ideal, 'a longing to become one with that ideal which lies outside the individual man or woman, apprehended as an intuitively sensed first principle'. The unattainability of that becoming one, the inadequacy of his own 'I', is the perpetual source of Man's dissatisfaction and pain (Tarkovsky 1986, 1987). This artistic striving he associates with the search for both beauty and the spiritual, and he distinguishes it from the other 'embodiment of the creative human spirit' science, in that science discovers and art creates. Tarkovsky acknowledges, as have many others, the place of intuition in science. 'At the moment of scientific discovery, logic is replaced by intuition', which he identifies as a way of thinking, compared with intuition in art, where, 'as in religion, intuition is tantamount to conviction, to faith. It is a state of mind, not a way of thinking'. In film after film, Tarkovsky explores memory and its relationship to reality and relationships, most vividly in *Solaris* (1973), from the novel by Stanislau Lem (1961) and in *Mirror* (1974) and *Nostalgia* (1981), (Turovskaya, 1989). Reality and morality against a historical background are central themes in *Andre Rublev* (1972) and *Stalker* (1979), and in the latter the central protagonist is represented as a Holy Fool handling wishes and disillusionment for his clientele in a mysterious dislocated landscape. The point I want to make is not only about the films and their poetry, but how art, in this case cinematic poetry, takes up psychological threads and weaves them into an aspect of culture which informs and sustains consciousness.

Art, society, politics

Camille Paglia set a cat among the pigeons with her *Sexual Personae* (2001), which went like a noisy lawnmower through many conventions, including the new Establishment feminism. In the Beginning, she begins, was nature, with human life beginning – as Jack London (1908) described it – in flight and fear. An emerging civilisation (and by implication I assume the mind that accompanies and develops from it) required a state of illusion, with 'the idea of the ultimate benevolence of nature and God (being) the most potent of man's survival mechanisms' (Paglia 2001). With Freud, more or less, Paglia says that sexuality and eroticism are to be found where nature and culture meet, or clash. My own perspective on this is that raw sexuality and aggression and the propensity to chase and take and bite and eat are there before mind, and both excitingly and troublingly shape and colour the emerging mind. But the emerging mind – still emerging, I think – is in turn washed through with the prevailing culture, with the products of other people's experience and imagination, from individualistic experiments in anarchic art to occasional big and institutionalised programmes as in totalitarian State Art as under the Nazi and Soviet regimes. But we also see such influences in the unstoppable and ever-widening torrent of yarns, folk stories, pop music, drama, film and TV, theatre and literature great and small, *all of it* starting out in small back rooms where individual brains and minds (not uncommonly with personal problems to project and sort out, as biography after biography shows) cast about to 'reach', as it's often put, other minds, to 'raise their awareness', 'shock', 'persuade' or 'provoke'.

Art is powerful. But for whose good? Anne Glyn-Jones, in 'Holding up a Mirror' (1996), shows how the arts play their part in reflecting, moulding, amplifying, encouraging and promoting social developments which in turn, of course, influence the arts and so on in a cycle that, while it can be virtuous, can also presage the collapse of civilisations, for example in Greece and Rome, where increasing violence and depravity (or permissiveness) in the theatre accompanied social and cultural decline. But which came first? The Roman chronicler Orosius warned those who complained about how things were going to the dogs that 'they should blame the theatres and not the times' (Glyn-Jones 1996). Certainly the *rise* and reinforcement of civilisations owes much to the arts too. There are the wonders of the cinema and of million-pound firework displays now, but the construction of cathedrals was a miracle too, as they towered phenomenally and beautifully above landscapes, villages and towns, begging the question what kind of beings were they who – over several hundred years – built them. People living in one- and two-roomed cottages could not fail to feel full of awe at the art, the building and the boldness and organisation involved; just as evolutionists speculate that the glory of the peacock in the eyes of the peahen is how well-endowed in genes if not in genitals the male DNA-donor must be, to have all that spare capacity for decoration beyond the necessities of mere individual survival.

End point

What would our earliest, near-human ancestors have been like to meet? Perhaps someone like a Bonobo chimpanzee, a kind of early holy fool (perhaps even an eccentric outsider in the tribe) who we might catch painting and able to exchange some kind of communication with us; who might even have a tale to tell, one that, given a million or two years, might be recognisable as one of our myriad cultural myths, perhaps one in a version currently being distributed on DVDs? There is no reason to suppose that the basic, archetypal mind, down to its roots in the neural network and the unconscious, has changed much over millions of years; consciousness, however, is still unfolding from it, as old mind speaks to new mind across space and time, new minds generate art, and art continues to shape and expand consciousness.

9

Connecting up

On making up one's mind

Self-awareness

The clue is in the wording. The nature of the sense of 'I' at the centre of consciousness is not only conceptually elusive but challenges satisfactory definition too, because again and again we find ourselves falling back on tautology, the description of something in terms of itself. McCrone (1990) is one of the relatively few who specify the problem of 'the shadowy "self" lurking in the background of the mind that remains even after we have stripped away all our thoughts and feelings'. 'Self awareness', he says, 'is a tricky piece of mental footwork – learning to turn awareness around on itself and then living with the net of memories created by this feat.' This however is the point: our sense of self grows out of having more than one self which – to anticipate the kind of model I am going to use – is like a kind of acrobatic act of identical-seeming performers in which there is the illusion of there always being *someone* in the air.

Some intriguing accounts of consciousness based on neural function, for example Jaynes (1976), Popper and Eccles (1977), Hofstadter (1979), Humphrey (1984), Edelman (1987, 1989), Dennett (1990, 1997), Penrose (1990, 1994), Gazzaniga (1994), Crick (1994), Chalmers (1996), Pinker (1997), Ramachandran and Blakeslee (1998), and Damasio (2000), suggest, albeit in rather different ways, the need for two or more kinds of minds, that is within the same brain, for the task of generating a sense of 'I'. However even these comprehensive accounts don't quite grasp the nettle of describing a psychological mechanism for the task. I will select some of the suggestions they put forward where they seem to fit in with my own attempt at a neuropsychological model for a self-conscious mind.

First, I will outline the main topics I have described so far as the parts for this jigsaw puzzle; and later discuss how they could be locked together *and* into some aspects of brain function which are thought to underwrite consciousness.

Constituents of consciousness

1 *Art, artefact, creativity*
   Throughout human evolution, human history, cultural development and our individual development we receive and make stories and images about ourselves and the world. From the greatest of the arts and monuments to the furnishings of everyday life we exist in a sea of perceptions, imagery, symbolism and language which arise from within, consciously and unconsciously; and from without, again, as we have seen, not always with our full awareness; and whether from within or without, constantly mediated and modified by an active, creative, memory-laden, rationalising and fantasising mind. To emphasise this, because it is largely neglected in the literature of consciousness, I would describe it as if the whole of the arts wash through raw, basic awareness and give it colour, value, diversity and depth.

2 *Archetype*
   The above circular process – art feeding mind, and mind feeding personal and public creativity and productivity, which then re-cycles to mind, has deep roots in both sides. Evolutionary necessity has laid down in us the neural potentiality to perceive in our cultures, and to project *into* our cultures, the very archetypal symbols, imagery and narratives the human species has itself created, which as individuals we therefore recognise, and on which our consciousness depends. This is a key notion – the extent to which memory is inner re-cognition. To continue our marine metaphor, it is as if the symbolic nutrient fluid in which we are suspended is itself constantly sustained and renewed by a deeper, earthier, more biological culture.

3 *Philosophies of imagination and reality*
   The politics and social expectations of culture and of all kinds and degrees of cooperation and conflict lead us to draw on private fantasies and public mythologies (for example about authority, acceptance and acquiescence) alike to make sense, make our way and get our way. This applies as much to the living of ordinary lives as it does to the development and implementation of grand ideologies and their symbolic trappings, and the whole panoply

and variety of religious and philosophical belief. These take up the (relatively) innocent arts-based ideas and beliefs, and render them communal, whether in small communities, liberal societies or tightly controlled tyrannies – e.g. as flags, uniforms, symbols and style. This represents, as it were, the *realpolitik* of psychology.

4   *Attachment theory, the unconscious and the necessities, demands and scope of relationships*
How does all this culture-bound, imaginative, abstract stuff get into the brain? The social and cultural context, from the earliest and simplest to the latest and most complex, is hard-wired out of evolutionary necessity, because the almost unique helplessness of human infants makes several years of help from experienced adults essential afterwards; the infant must attract help from adults and the social group *and* use it competently. Those that survive had the skills of the attachment dynamic in them from birth, and hence this cluster of capacities became part of the innate repertoire of the species. The development of our big brains that made biologically premature birth (i.e. small overall size) necessary, and required competent attachment behaviour, also equipped us with the cerebral capacity (memory, language, imagery, fantasy, anticipation, insight) to handle relationships within that developing attachment, and to be empathic, deceptive, self-deceptive and manipulative – i.e. political – and potentially paranoid as well as potentially loving, caring, creative, altruistic and *trusting* about others – a curious yet essential component of social cohesion and sanity which Ridley (1996) successfully traces all the way from the sometimes misunderstood 'selfish' gene. But with this awareness of self and others came apprehension and guilt too – the 'what ifs' of life, and conscience, because what as an animal we could do without thinking, such as sex and murder in the tribe and in the family (Freud 1950), now generated reflection and empathy, excuses, rationalisation, explanation, myth and neurosis. Because it isn't feasible to attend to everything at once, especially such heated and mixed feelings about oneself in relation to others *and* stay sane and focused, great stretches and depths of feelings remained partly or wholly out of reach except, partially, in fantasies and dreams. The crowded machinery of the attachment dynamic and the new, imaginative, image-laden brain resulted in such inner feelings and the economy and efficiency of the attachment system to be largely out of the mind's eye.

5 *Evolution from chemistry and genes to brain and mind*
The outline above of the kinds of feelings human beings would have, some holding them back, others saying 'go', represents what happens when consciousness begins to dawn and illuminates raw awareness. We look at animals, from ants and snails and bees and birds to cats, horses and dogs, and think we see them seeking comfort and safety, food, safe places to be, even creature comforts, and even appearing to enjoy themselves in activity and play. Even single-celled creatures seem to seek A and avoid B, ingest X and eliminate Y, as if they knew something. Higher animals do, in a sense, but not with much if anything in the way of memory or anticipation or motivation. They just do it, no doubt with coarse arousal and emotion and pleasure at some unknowable, literally unimaginable level. They are not like us, however much we may, in our anthropomorphic way, wish it or will it; *it is we who are like them*; but with the crucial 'extra' of a potential awareness of animal tendencies that we largely prefer to remain potential. But animal instincts go beyond what monkeys do to each other. Each kind of animal life grows ultimately out of earlier forms, and while pioneering biologists and ethologists like Tinbergen (1951, 1953) and Lorenz (1977) argued coherently for a continuity all the way from the needs and behaviour of the lowest animals, including protozoa, through social life and culture to conceptual thought and language, this is also implicit in Freudian theory (Sulloway 1979). 'The learning of language', said Lorenz, 'is ... based on a phylogenetic programme which ensures that the child's innate power of abstract thought is integrated and reintegrated on every occasion with the vocabulary that belongs to its cultural tradition' (Lorenz 1977). This is a very long way from the amoeba in the drop of water, yet it is difficult to draw a convincing gulf between what it needs and the 'wants' we elaborate for ourselves in our culture, even if it is a pleasant bar near the pool rather than merely the brighter and warmer part of the puddle. Given good-enough brains and the fortunate accident of social conditions in which those big brains can survive and develop, consciousness begins to grow out of awareness and becomes aware of its substrate, the depths of the unconscious. And by being in a position *to be* aware of it we grow a conscious mind: another necessarily circular argument.

I do want to emphasise the point about animals, in the understanding of human consciousness: every time we attribute something human to another creature – even a microscopic protozoan 'heading' for something, or a woodlouse or worm 'trying to hide', a bird 'building' a nest, a crocodile 'taking care of' its young, a dog or cat being 'nice' to us, or a big cat being 'ferocious', the true situation is not that they are just like us but that we are like them – particularly in our unconscious minds, which, to varying degrees, is where the behaviour exists in the animals too. It is something which in this sense we share.

Where is the unconscious mind?

But first, where *from*? We inherit its foundations, as I have argued, from even the most primitive animals' responses to the exigencies of their lives, all the way back to single-celled protozoa. In this sense, the unconscious represents a kind of rich, multi-layered sediment of learning and experience very gradually shaped up, as we go up the animal world, by a dawning awareness. But this geological metaphor, useful as a means of getting a grip on the territory, is one we should leave behind; it is best not to be seduced by models of the mind which place the 'unconscious' as if in geological or hydrodynamic terms, heaving, surging, being 'contained', leaking and occasionally erupting from down below. Like all metaphors, this one can help or mislead, and was simply borrowed by the science of the time just as the notion of evil spirits served hundreds of years earlier, and metaphors from information technology more recently (Tyrer and Steinberg 2005). By the same token we should be cautious about models from quantum theory too, valuable though they are.

To an extent the unconscious mind represents electrochemical brain processes in nerves and synapses which enable thought, yet of which we are no more aware than we are of the activity in the cells of the kidney. That too is unconscious. Bohm, also a quantum physicist and philosopher, has described words and phrases as an archaeology of our thought processes, a metaphor which has moved on from the rocks towards art and culture, and suggests that within words there are hierarchies of meaning of which we cannot be aware all of the time (Bohm 1980; Steinberg 2004a). Ehrenzweig (1965) has related the ideas of gestalt theory (*gestalt*: shape, form) to the perception of the aesthetic: that there is an 'articulating tendency', noted also by William James and Sigmund Freud, that our minds tend to select for use and understanding accessible, relatively precise forms of perception while setting aside the vague and incoherent. But the material left behind, the background field or context, remains influential. Arnheim (1966, 1992) has discussed gestalt theory in relation to brain function, that which is perceived socially, culturally and aesthetically as a whole, being rather like the illusion of motion when a sequence of on–off lights gives an impression of words moving along a display, or like a rapid succession of stills on a film screen. Gestalt theory remains controversial, and perhaps has been applied too widely, but as applied to the psychology of art and culture one can see how words and symbols may be particularly effective because of the context they come from (e.g. someone speaking with the authority of an institution) without the recipient appreciating quite why. One thinks of the authority of a white-coated doctor in a hallowed clinical institution, even though he or she may be taking a clinic on their first day after qualification and know next to nothing: such things happen. On a similar note, architecture and building design may be more or less taken for granted, albeit mildly liked or disliked, but may be designed unconsciously to impress, reassure, or intimidate.

One model for the unconscious mind is that it exists in the interaction between nerve cells and words, but primarily in words and phrases and their cultural and personal gestalt (Steinberg 2004a); in other words, *it isn't actually there*, except as the availability of nerve cells like so many transistors, until a train of words and a shower of their possible, alternative, clear, vague, misunderstood and implied meanings, and the feelings they generate, begin to dip in and out of our conscious feelings and understanding. It is exactly like insinuation and innuendo sparking off meanings and meanings within meanings not only different in different members of the audience, but unanticipated and even unthought of by the speaker. I'm not sure how close this is to Pinker's conception of sequences in language (Pinker 1994, 1997).

The point is that instead of the 'unconscious' being a kind of cavern-like repository of imagery, feelings and meanings, it is more like an archetypal, elaborate linguistic mesh strung between the neural, the personal and the social for the 'I' to scramble across like a small spider in a vast web. This notion of the unconscious being 'out here', socially, verbally and culturally, as much as 'in there' has been argued by Luria (1976) and Vigotsky (e.g. Frawley 1997). It is taken further in a complex argument, outlined by Arnheim (1992), in which gestalt psychologists have argued links with the physical sciences, 'making it possible to coordinate the functioning of the mind with the organic and inorganic world as a whole'; thus 'the laws governing the functioning of the brain and, by extension, the physical universe in general, were assumed to be reflected in mental activity as well'. Now, I do not fully understand what the gestalt theorists are getting at, and I am not sure gestalt psychology as originally described, for example by Wertheimer in 1912 (discussed by Arnheim 1992), is complete enough for the task. But it may prove a conceptual vehicle, a kind of booster rocket, that takes us in the kind of direction that brings together physics, brain and mind as considered later in this chapter and in Chapter 11. Is part of our consciousness and memory 'stored' in the words, forms and rules of long-term memory of literature, for example? (*see* Otis (1994), and p. 164). Meanwhile, it raises the intriguing question that if the unconscious mind is not all there until caught, as if in a finely evolved and adapted linguistic net – which is not *quite* the same thing as saying we need words to think with, as this archetypal net fashions the words too – could consciousness also be a potentiality, a process, that depends on inner and outer symbols, metaphors and stimuli? Thus, consciousness doesn't sit there, like a psychological and neuronal receptacle waiting to be filled in and topped up – the flow of information from within and without *makes* that receptacle, renewing it all the time, so that the transient appears constant.

Appears constant to whom? We will come to that next.

The Self and the brain

For the Self we need the brain, though not only the brain. Karl Popper and John Eccles (1977) describe three worlds of the brain – physical, psychological and cultural, although in their book Eccles does propose the Self as something above and beyond what even neurological, psychological and psychosocial interaction can achieve. From time to time the idea of a self-aware Mind existing in the universe and picked up by the brain as receiver/transmitter has been floated, and I am not sure if that is exactly what Eccles means; but, in a sense, he gives at least the scientific part of the game away by saying that he *cannot believe* that conscious experience has no future after the body's death. Kenan Malik (2000) discusses human nature rather than consciousness, and leaves the 'I' as a given which, among other things, distinguishes man from animals and machines, to that extent showing the limits of a scientific explanation, and gives language and social relationships as that which makes us different from both.

Julian Jaynes (1976), as we have seen, proposed that the Self emerged out of one part of the brain hearing hallucinatory voices from the other. Douglas Hofstadter (1979) required 'sub-brains' or subsystems (of which the Self is one) for his 'shared' or 're-entrant' model, the terms borrowed from computer technology, and analogous to two (or more) 'timesharing' programs running on a single machine. Michael Gazzaniga (1994) proposes that consciousness depends on a huge, innate complexity in the brain which, in a process which only *looks like* learning, in fact represents the brain 'searching through its library of circuits and accompanying (behavioural and cognitive) strategies to match the enormously variable challenges of the environment' – which, for me, is a way of accounting in neurological terms for an essentially archetypal process (also see Goonatilake 1991). Francis Crick (1994), taking visual perception as his exemplar, suggests that synchronised firing of the neurones which connect the thalamus, a subcortical forebrain structure, one on each side and connected to each other, and which act as a relay for all senses except smell heading for the cortex, represents the neural correlate of consciousness. To function as such, what is known in neuroscience as 'binding', has to be achieved, that is the putting together in a coherent way all the different kinds of input – for example a friend's face, his expression as he speaks, what he says, and memories and thoughts about him. Crick gives a sophisticated account of awareness, attention and the mind, but still remains below the 'glass ceiling' of accounting for the observing 'I'. Steven Pinker, in a comprehensive account of the role of language in the human mind, is honest enough to say, while only a fifth of the way into his very big book, that the problem of self-awareness 'beats the heck out of me'; but, perhaps more helpfully than he realises, at least for my own model, he says:

> *it's just irrational to insist that sentience remains unexplained after all the manifestations of sentience have been accounted for, just because the computations don't have anything sentient in them. It's like insisting that wetness remains unexplained even after all the manifestations of wetness have been accounted for, because moving molecules aren't wet. (Pinker 1997)*

He is right, of course, in thus drawing attention to the flaws in reductionism and its inevitable disconnectedness.

VS Ramachandran and Sandra Blakeslee (1998) describe the 'zombie' phenomenon, popular at the moment in this field, which is the notion of complexly functioning minds in more or less normally behaving people who are not, indeed do not need to be, conscious. It is, of course, in the nature of a philosophical thought-experiment, and may be one way of coping with Pinker's, Crick's and others' frustration at all the ingredients for a fully functioning mind being explored in the most elaborate and sophisticated ways and *still* we can't identify the nature of consciousness. The sense of 'I' may be, they suggest, an illusion; but this is qualified by the suggestion that there is no single entity corresponding to self within the brain. It may be useful to have a sense of self, among our many selves (embodied, executive, passionate, etc.), and a useful idea for thinking about the brain, but 'when we achieve a more mature understanding (of mental life and neural processes) the word self may disappear from our vocabulary' (Ramachandran and Blakeslee 1998). So there it is, consciousness as a kind of useful if slightly neurotic fixation; which leads me to think that we're getting somewhere.

The body and the mind: duels and dualists

Before discussing Dennett's, Edelman's and Damasio's models for consciousness, a brief diversion into some philosophical views may help set the scene. The apparent need for the components of a self-generating mind to require dual explanation within psychobiology sets it apart from the dualism of René Descartes (1596–1650) that consciousness, occupying no space, therefore owes nothing to the material world and cannot originate in the body; instead, as the 'I' or the soul, is completely distinct. John Searle (1997) reminds us that dualism is by no means outdated or intellectually discredited, and provides a useful classification. At the same time he indicates a new dualism, the difference between what most people believe – that we have a body and a mind or soul – and the views of most philosophers, psychologists, cognitive scientists and neurobiologists working on consciousness. As outlined in Chapter 6, Searle divides those who think about the matter into *monists* who maintain that the world is made of only one kind of stuff, and *dualists* who see mind and body as fundamentally different. *Monists* subdivide into idealists who think everything is mental, and materialists who think everything is physical. *Dualists* subdivide into 'substance dualists' who believe the terms mind and body identify two different kinds of substances, and 'property dualists' who think the same material or substance – human beings – can have two kinds of property at the same time, i.e. mental and physical.

Searle goes on to discuss the position of David Chalmers which represents another kind of duality. Chalmers argues that the materialist position (much of the most influential of which leans towards analogies with computer technology) gives an acceptable account of the mind up to but excluding consciousness; he says 'consciousness arises from functional organisation' – i.e. the way neurones function, with or without computer analogies – 'but it is not a functional state' (Chalmers, 1996). Searle refutes this position in an exchange with Chalmers worth reading, and gives Chalmers' response that, whatever we think of neuronal activity, to say that 'the brain causes consciousness', whatever the brain mechanisms (so far) described, is inadequate, and that there needs to be – if I follow the argument correctly – both conscious and non-conscious processes, the former coming from beyond the physical operations of the brain as conventionally described, and in this context floats the idea that consciousness, or elements of consciousness, could be (Chalmers doesn't assert that they *are*) an information-bearing property inherent in all matter in the universe, called panpsychism (Chalmers 1996; Searle 1997).

Roger Penrose (1990, 1994), who is a mathematician and quantum theorist, rises above and beyond trying to relate what the brain might do to what consciousness might be (which on reflection seems fair enough when framed that way), and his argument is complex. He sees mathematics and quantum physics as having an explanatory potential for consciousness that neither neurobiology nor computer science can reach, and uses Godel's theorem (Hofstadter 1979) of the incomplete nature of mathematics; and, using Penrose's conclusion about the theorem rather than his mathematical explanation (despite his persuasive words that it is pretty straightforward), he states not only that mathematical rules of proof remain insufficient to prove even arithmetic, but that such computational rules cannot account for consciousness (and such elements as intuition and insight). Penrose identifies as a key issue aesthetics – the perception and appreciation of art – as representing a capacity for awareness of absolutes in the Platonic sense (*see* p. 106). 'Might it be the case that our awareness is somehow able to make contact with such absolutes, and it is *this* [Penrose's italics] that gives consciousness its essential strength?' (Penrose 1994). But even more than Penrose's position on aesthetics as above and beyond neurobiology *and* computer science, his supposition is that the physics of *quantum indeterminism* may be a vital component in the fact and exercise of free will in particular and consciousness generally. To put quantum indeterminism at its simplest, but I think correctly, this means that quantum particles can be put into the *superposition* of being in two places at the same time. This, I am assured by an astrophysicist friend, to whom such matters are bread and butter, is not just supposition on paper but, as every modern physicist knows, experimentally demonstrable (Speer 2006, personal communication). The binding problem (*see* p. 146) by which separate perceptions are perceived in their entirety could be explained by quantum processes within the brain, and here Penrose invokes gravity, more specifically *gravitational OR*. This is gravitational objective reduction, a mathematical proposition that two states can become a single one of the two states on a calculable time scale, and that this could be demonstrated experimentally (Penrose 2004). But for the brain to achieve such pyrotechnics, something far more elaborate than neuronal signalling would be needed, for example the neuronal microtubules, which are found as cell constituents all the way back to single-celled organisms without nervous systems. This could explain the ability of single-celled organisms like the amoeba (*see* pp. 54,103, 185) to learn; at which point we are, comparatively speaking, approaching the basic biology with which we started out (*see* pp. 54–6) and very near to some of the biological fundamentals of Freudian theory (*see* p. 54). Penrose argues that this could mean that each individual neurone could itself have its own microtubular nervous system; and this astronomical complexity could support activity describable and explicable in quantum terms (Penrose 1994, 2004).

Nicholas Humphrey, theoretical psychologist, provides some of the most accessible reading about the unlimited complexities of the subject, and unlike many authorities he worries away at the core question of 'I' and self rather than gliding over or dismissing it. He argues, as I did earlier (*see* p. 31), that experience requires an experiencer, and – contemplating the emergence of a sense of self in a baby – suggests (while wondering if the idea is bizarre) that Self could be composed of several or many selves. He quotes from Marcel Proust's *Swann's Way* in his *Remembrance of Things Past* where, waking in the middle of the night, Proust doesn't at first know who he is or where he is, and feels only a 'rudimentary sense of existence, such as may lurk and flicker in the depths of an animal's consciousness' (Humphrey 2002). Perhaps we have all had such experiences, if not on waking, then perhaps when intoxicated in one way or another.

Once again there is the suggestion, or perhaps it is an argument born of frustration with the elusive sense of self, that however one tries one cannot escape a kind of within-the-mind dualism, that of the observer and the observed. This will be central to my own model for the self-conscious mind, and we will come back to it after looking at some feasible neurological and neurophilosophical models that would partially support such a position.

Dennett, Edelman and Damasio

These three authors, a philosopher, a neuroscientist and a neurologist – among other things, as those who venture into consciousness tend to be – have written so extensively that I cannot hope to even outline here all the twists and turns of their arguments. Instead, keeping to my theme of how proto-self might observe proto-self and become 'I', I will extract what seems to me the bare essence of their accounts and use them in my model for Brain, Mind and the sense of Self.

Daniel Dennett, philosopher, provides in numerous publications a most engaging, important and impressive account of Mind, minds and a mind, but not, I feel in my bones, *the* mind. He too has enjoyed a prolonged disputation with Searle (1997). His conceptual model is essentially drawn from computational neuroscience, and he seems to doubt the true existence of qualia (subjective perceptions and feelings about them) and consciousness itself, by which I presume he means that his model doesn't account for them. What I want to draw out from Dennett's model is his key concept of *multiple drafts*, which he contrasts with the 'Cartesian Theatre', a supposed arena in the brain or mind where all kinds of memories and perceptions come together and where consciousness is forged. The Multiple Drafts Model proposes that 'all varieties of thought or mental activity are accomplished by parallel, multitrack processes of interpretation and elaboration of sensory inputs' (Dennett 1991) all under continuous 'editorial revision', and happening all over the brain. Dennett doesn't deny the phenomenon of narrative, but it is a constantly edited, re-edited narrative. There is no single, final narrative, which Dennett dismisses, dismissing the stream of consciousness, which would be a coterminous phenomenon, along with it. I think Dennett's model takes us along a useful route, away from the 'Cartesian Theatre' (which reminded me of the 'homunculus' notion, of an observer sitting inside the brain, and which only pushes the mystery back a notch), but perhaps in the direction of my own model, the Cinema: all of it, best boys, gaffers, accountants, technologists, projectionists, scriptwriters, stars, audiences, advertising, myths and all, and especially the myths.

Edelman (1987, 1989, 2005) provides a particularly compelling neural account of consciousness, or at least of its essential substrate. Edelman refers to his theory as Neural Darwinism because the brain has to deal with, contains and selects from enormous variation (as Penrose said, more than neurones could possibly handle, *see* pp. 148–9); indeed there is so much information and information-processing, at all levels from the molecular upwards, and with such constant and plastic variation from task to task and person to person, that neither evolution nor a computer model of the mind could have devised sufficient error-correcting codes (hence, perhaps, Dennett's continuous editing model). Nor, Edelman maintains, could a computer handle it, because the information to work on is variable and dynamically interchanging and the *context* constantly changes. How does the brain do it? Edelman proposes a three-part theory of neuronal group selection. First, *developmental selection*, guided by genetic inheritance, by which millions of variant patterns of connections between nerve cells, that is, at synaptic level, develop during the earliest stages of neuroanatomical development within each area of the brain. This gives each area a repertoire of millions of variant circuits or neuronal groups. Second, *experiential selection*, building upon developmental selection, modifies these neuronal groups by favouring some and weakening others, in the light of environmental stimuli, 'subject to the constraints of value systems' by which Edelman refers to 'rewards and responses necessary to survival' (Edelman, 2005). Third, *re-entry*, or the development of large numbers of reciprocal connections between brain areas locally and over long distances, thus creating a map of connected brain areas which are coordinated over space and time – i.e. which handle what happens when. Crucial to the theory is the notion of degeneracy, which in this context means the ability of structurally different elements of a system to perform the same function, 'a ubiquitous biological property' requiring complexity at genetic, cellular, organisational and population levels, and a central feature of immune responses; it is the ultimate in belt and braces. The resulting complexity, plasticity and ability enables the brain to cope adaptively with enormous complexity, diversity and change. Within this there is a 'dynamic core', centred on the thalamocortical system (*see* p. 146) which has a fast-acting, millisecond by millisecond, re-entrant structure which is largely self-contained ('it speaks mainly to itself') and provides an enormously elaborate non-conscious system that sub-serves conscious systems, for example by enabling binding (*see* p. 149) to happen and relating value-category memory (e.g. 'what I like') to perceptual categories (e.g. kittens, trees). Edelman distinguishes *primary consciousness*, which he describes as equivalent to animal awareness, unaccompanied by 'any sense of a socially defined self with a concept of a past or a future', from *higher order consciousness*, the ability to be 'conscious of being conscious' i.e. the ability to reconstruct what Edelman describes as the 'remembered present'. This means the ability to construct a conscious scene in a fraction of a second. (I would say *reconstruct* a scene.) Edelman describes this as an integrated awareness of multiple sensation, 'perceptions, images, thoughts, emotions, vague feelings and so on', with 'all past experience engaged in forming my integrated awareness of this single moment' and requires perception of other selves, through social interaction (Edelman 2005). All this gives higher order consciousness power in the original Darwinian sense, enabling the management of complex environments (including social environments and ideas about other people's thinking, *see* pp. 84,85). In evolutionary terms, comparative neural anatomy suggests that primary consciousness (animal awareness) appeared at the transition between reptiles on the one hand and birds and mammals on the other. Again, I see a necessarily circular argument embedded here: to develop a sense of self one must somehow form an inner, value-laden image of another's self. But to know what to recognise there must be some kind of imagery of self to begin with. But that's all right, as we shall see.

This is only an outline of Edelman's account, which should be read, but I have selected elements which straddle neuroanatomy and neurological theory, aspects of the philosophy of consciousness and evolution and which seem to me consistent with several other people's models of the conscious mind, including the one that follows.

Antonio Damasio, neurologist, also provides a model based on neuroanatomical structures. Like Edelman's and Dennett's his argument is elaborate and involved and does not lend itself to summary. Damasio states the need to divide the problem of consciousness into two parts: what he calls the 'movie in the brain' of multiple sensory images (visual, auditory, olfactory and so on), and the means of developing a sense of ownership of it. He describes a number of selves, beginning with the *proto-self*, which is a preconscious, biological collection of neural patterns located throughout the nervous system and concerned with regulating the internal state of the organism. This proto-self, Damasio emphasises, has no powers of perception and 'holds no knowledge'. It is not in one place but represents a dynamic (i.e. interactive, constantly changing) property of the nervous system.

It is the precursor to the *core self*, which Damasio (2000) describes as 'the transient protagonist of consciousness, generated for any object that provokes the core consciousness mechanism'. *Core consciousness* is the brain's non-verbal, inner representation 'of how the organism's own state is affected by the organism's processing of an object, and when this process enhances the image of the causative object, placing it saliently in a spatial and temporal context' (Damasio 2000). Now that is quite a statement to absorb, but it repays attention. I would say that much the same has been said, sometimes more clearly but often less so, in the psychoanalytic theory known as object relations, where 'object' means that towards which action or desire is directed. I would simplify it as a statement, again a circular one, in which the observer makes more of himself by making something of the *other's* effect on *him*; which brings about change in the observer, who then makes more of what he perceives. To me this is a raw statement of the bedrock of proto-love and proto-hate, such as an amoeba with insight and feeling could develop; it also reverberates with the quantum notion so many 'objective' observers have trouble with – that the observer changes what he or she observes.

The third category in Damasio's schema is the *autobiographical self*, which requires the existence of the core self and core consciousness, and is 'based on permanent but dispositional –' (i.e. not always active, but available) '– records of core self experiences' (2000). The autobiographical self consists of memory of the past and anticipation of the future, and sets of memory about identity can be reactivated as both neural pattern and image whenever needed; it is the Self. Dispositions are described by Damasio in complex organisms as representing:

> *large repertoires of knowledge, the possibility of choosing among many available responses, the ability to construct novel combinations of response and the ability to plan ahead ... a substantial part [of them] must be provided by the genome and be innate ... the control of emotions is part of this dispositional stock. (Damasio 2000, p.139)*

Enlarging on dispositions in relation to memory, Damasio describes them as:

> *records which are dormant and implicit rather than active and explicit, as images are ... [they are] not only records of the sensory aspects of the object ... but also records of the motor adjustments that*

> *necessarily accompanied the gathering of the sensory signals ... and records of the obligate emotional reaction to the object. (Damasio 2000, p.160)*

I believe that Damasio is describing the same idea as Jungian archetypes.

For the proto-self to operate in generating the autobiographical self it requires, according to Damasio's model, a neural base for itself, one for representing the 'causative object' – i.e. that which the core self registers, and 'at least one other structure which *re-presents* both proto-self and proto-self modified by its object' (2000). Hence there needs to be what Damasio calls a second order neural pattern to generate a second order and enhanced map of the object. 'This succession of such re-presentations constitutes a neural pattern that becomes ... the basis for an image ... of a relationship between object X and the proto-self changed by X' (2000).

Both Damasio and Edelman use the term imagery in the sense of an internal representation of the outside world, although I prefer to distinguish between a coarse and *relatively* simple representation of the outside world, such as a bee might have in dealing with fields and gardens in relation to a hive, or a domestic cat might have of a house and its environs, and a multi-sensory inner picture to which are attached multiple possible memories, multiple possible anticipations and fantasies, and multiple and quite probably conflicting feelings.

Damasio also coins the particularly interesting phrase 'something-to-be-known', distinguishing between an object registering on the proto-self, or *being*, with the re-presentation of object, organism (= observer) and their relation to each other, which is the beginning of *knowing*.

Connecting up

The study of consciousness is not at a stage where one can regard all the authorities on the subject, past and present, as working on the same thing, as when several European countries make an aircraft – the wings here, the fuselage there, the engines somewhere else and so on. An attempt to stitch other people's models together too assiduously would produce something like Frankenstein's monster. Instead, I am more concerned with finding concepts that seem to be consistent enough with each other for connections to be made between them in the construction of a model for the self-conscious mind; interpreting from A to B, rather than attempting precise translations. Several of these potential connections between conceptions of consciousness have already been indicated.

First I would like to remind the reader of some of the necessary building techniques.

1   The concept of the *dynamic*; that most steady states in biology and psychology are the outcome of competing influences.
2   The concept of *levels of organisation*, from the outward appearances through biological, psychological, behavioural, social and cultural processes affecting appearances, with an influential *unconscious* as one of the levels.
3   The concept that consciousness, Self and accompanying behaviour is at any moment on a dual sliding scale of (a) *personality development* to date and (b) *circumstances*. In a crisis, for example, one person may behave more maturely and another more childishly, for example with a tantrum, and their position, with one foot on each scale, will affect (1) and (2). But regression, as psychoanalysts would call a retrospective move to an earlier state (the very word sounds like a reproof) is a capacity best disconnected from immaturity or disorder, although it can explain aspects of both. To operate as if child-like is usually distinguished from being 'childish', and although there could be a better word for it, the term also conveys something positive about curiosity, creative apperception, receptivity, appreciation and productivity. This is taken up in point 6 on page 161.
4   The importance of *metaphor*, not only because for explanatory purposes metaphors provide familiar analogies to help describe the unfamiliar, but because *that* is also fundamental to the way we think and use language. Words are symbols of things – they are analogues of one sort or another from the start. Indeed, 'from the start' and 'fundamental' are metaphors. Our consciousness and our thinking are layered metaphors, from words and symbols through archetypes, narratives and our autobiographical, self-affirming accounts of ourselves.

A mechanism for Io, the Observing I, in six stages

1 Where Dennett mentions the 'Cartesian Theatre' in the mind, in order to dismiss it, and Damasio the 'movie in the mind', I will use as my example the mind in the movie, from studio to cinema.

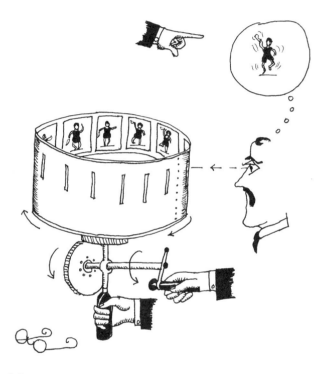

Figure 9.1

Watching a film requires among many other things a marriage between the technology of the cinema and way the eye and brain works, so that a succession of still pictures separated by a shuttering system and at the right speed produces a smoothly moving image. Various devices which date from early experiments with moving pictures, some of them now available as toys, show the phenomenon even more simply: looking through one of the slots in the cylinder drawn above (*see* Figure 9.1), while a succession of slightly different images rotate within, the observer sees for example a realistic running or jumping figure. Now, Damasio would rightly say that a model like this, whether a toy or the most sophisticated presentation imaginable, lacks ownership – a sense of Self which is, so to speak, making the running. To take a step in this direction, I am going to place my 'I' – and indeed my eye – *in* the box, as one of the still images of the figure. If that is mind-bending and perhaps logic-bending too, then given the magical creativity and display of Io production, that is perhaps how it has to be. Now, we will hold the model there for the moment and go to the mind and brain.

2   Within the spectrum of life, and despite the elusiveness of self-consciousness, it is not difficult to imagine a creature or for that matter a machine which registers the outside world and responds to it. A thermostat or an intruder alarm does this, and, taking a great leap, and perhaps being somewhat disrespectful to the wonders of life, I suggested that a spider responding to a fly in its web is also performing unconscious register–response behaviour. I would say it is aware, but not conscious in the sense of what we are exploring.

3   It is not clear in what sense a newborn baby is conscious. It 'looks' conscious like any small animal (like a spider in its web) demonstrates an aware responsiveness, though when we cast our minds back most people can't recall much before the age of about two or three years at the earliest, and even then it isn't clear that what we remember are experiences or events at the time or vague and perhaps inaccurate memories of them a little time later, perhaps reinforced by what we were told about falling out of the pram or whatever. But, for the moment, I am going to assume that in the human infant, even one that could turn out to be a Shakespeare or an Einstein, we start out with an aware, responsive, human animal without a sense of 'I', 'self' or identity. However, as we have seen, it has the most extraordinary inbuilt potential to develop one. The child's parents will have already begun to think about the child's possible name, and indeed what he or she 'will be like'. The stage could not be more set for the machinery of identification and self-identification to swing into highly efficient, highly acculturalised, well-tried action.

4   Here I want to produce, as if out of a hat, Jacques Lacan (1901–1981), French psychoanalyst and philosopher, whose writings are famed for their difficulty, indeed obscurity, and which, the reader needs to know, are highly controversial. However, being one who believes that people who contribute great ideas to knowledge may well be ordinary, fallible mortals whose life-work consists of a few precious diamonds amid vast quantities of excavated mud and

rubble (I would say this of Freud and Jung, for example), I think Lacan gave us two ideas about the mind and its development that would repay more attention. First, he saw the unconscious mind not as a great cauldron of instincts and drives but as a system of linguistic signifiers, a signifier being something conveying meaning, the precursor of words and language rather than formed words themselves. My own image of an unconscious and then conscious mind emerging from biological animal awareness would be rather like clusters of primitive meaning and feeling taking gradual shape as clusters of names, words and metaphors: sounds with meaning and feeling attached – like 'mama' and 'dada' – and an awareness – perhaps initially an 'animal' awareness – of the joy on the faces of parental figures who say 'she's talking about me!'. In my model, it is an evolutionary necessity, a *sine qua non* of survival, that the child comes equipped, innately, with the capacity to register signifiers and to connect with potentially responsive, ultimately caring figures as a complex human instinct. I would describe these as archetypal phenomena.

Second, Lacan introduced the idea of the mirror phase of development. (Mirrors are mysterious: not many people know why we see ourselves reversed from side to side in their reflection, yet not upside down.) Lacan, noting the prematurity and helplessness of the human infant and its need to make the beginning of a contribution to making its way in the world, decided on mimicry as a widespread ethological phenomenon that in the human infant would manifest, usefully, as *identification with something outside*. At this stage, we come upon another necessarily circular argument: at the earliest dawning of consciousness the infant doesn't know about 'inside' and 'outside', 'me' and 'you' – all that has yet to come. But, if Lacan was correct in seeing identification with something outside as an evolutionary necessity, the emergence of a notion of 'other' would set the scene for the emergence of 'self', with the cluster of feelings and meanings about self beginning to take some shape as a kind of silhouette against a cluster of feelings and meanings about 'other'. At this stage we are still talking about 'self' as a third-person phenomenon – we have yet to introduce a mechanism for ownership of this 'I'. We are also, I think, quite close to the statement of Antonio Damasio (*see* p. 153), the one I thought difficult but worth persisting with, and which describes proto-self 'at the inaugural instant' of sensing an object and immediately becoming modified by it. We therefore have the beginnings of a model for a self taking shape by identifying with what is not-self.

This argument is of the type I identified early in this book as illustrating the importance of taking nothing for granted in examining the nature of consciousness. Much child psychology has been discussed in terms of the infant being aware of this, doing that, then the parent does that, and so on, but all of this, it seems to me, is already well along the consciousness road. But why should an infant even take the slightest notice of the outside world, still less want to move about in it and do something with it – even merely grasping something – unless it had evolved-in, survival-enabling equipment that made such moves both possible and worth doing? Fortunately, amoeba-like, it comes equipped to move about, reach for, grab, ingest and do other things with what's outside for the sake of what's within. Of course, it has also had millions of years of adaptation and development to do such things so much better than an amoeba, or even a primate; for example, gazing at a face as if knowingly, and with a charming smile. But 'it' does this without knowing that it does.

5   *Components for the model for the experience of 'I' – Io.*
I will try to make the following account as direct and straightforward as I can; all the complexities and controversies are in the preceding chapters. The model is dependent on one not-yet-fully-conscious self becoming aware of another not-yet-fully-conscious self. When one self is aware of itself, you have the beginnings of an 'I'. But, somehow, these two selves have to be subjectively perceived as being in the same time and place; self aware of and observing itself, = Io.

But how to get there? We need:

(a) Animal awareness, which I have identified as inner, unconscious, evolved representations of the outside world, for example of the spider and its web and prey, all the way through to reptiles, birds and mammals. I will call this the animal self (AS).

(b) A new, proto-human brain which is able to handle complex perceptions from *within* as well as without, and which has evolved because of the evolutionary necessity of using and handling mutual relationships competently enough – as described in attachment theory. Without such competence (which ultimately includes inner reflection, handling ambiguity, sifting fantasy from reality, 'taking in' what is useful from outside and projecting out complicated hypotheses about the outside world and its denizens) – no survival and no advanced self. I will call this the cultural self (CS). It is not yet a sense of 'I'; as some have suggested, humanity could work, socially, on a 'zombie' basis, with no real sense of self-consciousness being necessary.

(c) A *teacher* (the caretaker, or parent, on the other side of the attachment dynamic) which feeds the dependent creature's animal self not just literally but with stimuli and provocations (e.g. how the AS represents and handles within itself the teacher's controlling tendencies). It 'feeds in' the requirements of the environment – proximity, safety, shelter, exploration, etc. Thus it deals with the local mini-culture – but is still no more than another animal self – AS. Hence we have two animal selves, one nurturing, the other being nurtured, but neither of them self-conscious in the sense used in this book.

(d) The neural potentiality to form, within, hard-wired archetypes. Minds/brains which are better at registering and retaining useful internal models of the outside culture (e.g. recognising and working with an effective parental figure) are more likely to survive, reproduce and become the kind of minds we know.

Through the capacity to *learn*, and the capacity to accumulate *archetypes* (an inner store of cultural instincts), the AS develops a CS. Both AS and CS are things the newly evolved proto-human brain can do. AS and CS are not co-terminous, and neither are conscious.

(e) *Memory*. The key to storage and useful disposal of what is stored is memory. As we have seen, memory isn't simply an internal record or archive, it is an active process (e.g. Rose 1993), operating *now* (not 'then') and which sifts and sorts past experience of cognitions and feelings in relation to future fantasies and anticipations. You cannot have, for example, a fear or fantasy of what mother will do next without present awareness of something she has stimulated already.

(f) A key tripartite constituent is simply the way things work – the physical and chemical laws of the universe – time, space and neural circuitry. Neural circuitry includes *delay* – the micro-split seconds needed for the brain anatomy and chemistry to register things and, after a brief refractory period, carry on registering things. We live our psychological lives a few milliseconds in the past. This fact of neural life operates in my 'toy cinema' model like the shutter – the split second gap between events that defines them. On the subject of space, remember that despite my 'tin can' cylindrical model this too is a metaphor – the brain operates holistically, not like a phrenological head.

(g) Finally, I am going to invoke the fairground again, because the above constituents of the model aren't spinning in space; AS within, AS without and the emergent CS within operate in a wider environment. We have already acknowledged such environments as primaeval ooze, forests and savannah, caves, cathedrals and city parks, all the way to sophisticated culture-generators like the arts, in the broadest sense, and exemplified by the cinema. I will suggest the fairground as a kind of compromise between earthiness and high art, with its mixture of art, craft, glamour, illusion, self-deception, playfulness and danger, its participants, colour and noise, and just on the periphery of that mirocosm, its own external and sustaining laws and machinery – of commerce, of folk culture, of community, of cables and generators.

6   *How does it all work?* Even with all this elaborate equipment, we still have only awareness, not consciousness. To develop a sense of 'I' the two internal, aware selves have to be both *distinct* (so that one can be aware of the other) and yet *in the same place* (so that self can be aware of self in the same time and place). These seem impossible requirements – separate but in the same place; though it does seem that quantum particles can achieve that. So it may be that we are at the impossible nucleus of the argument – perhaps a kind of psychic singularity or event horizon.

The AS is, I think, not hard to conceptualise. We have no difficulty with the spider's inner representation of its web, or the cat's of its home. What the CS registers is something outside its self – what I have called the caretaker, parent or teacher: There is something out there – an unidentified identity. The concept is still with us, from all degrees of religious belief, through mythology, to the art and culture of science fiction. The CS can be seeded (from outside) just as the AS is already rooted, in the fertile soil of the proto-human nervous system, with its complex capabilities and potentialities as described by Dennett, Edelman and Damasio (p. 150 *et seq.*) But, within the nervous system, it is somewhere else.

AS reflects CS like a mirror. It (and it is still only an 'it') registers that which is outside (an 'entity') looking in, and that which is inside, looking out, but the two sets of perceptions are still in different places, rather like two different animals, one contemplating feeling hungry, and another animal contemplating a rustling sound which might be a meal. Or like two different people each contemplating a rainbow. There is still the remaining split, an impassable glass barrier between awareness and self-awareness.

So, I will postulate an aspect of memory; that the back of our glass is silvered, like a mirror; but not merely a coat of something reflective, rather a complex, micro-thin coat of memory-retaining and anticipatory-generating neurochemistry, perhaps operating along the lines of something like 'e' (electronic) paper: an holistic function in the brain which holds imagery for long enough for it to become fixed and elaborated as imagination. By 'long enough' I mean milliseconds, and it holds the image for long enough and vividly enough to retain a fading reflection of the other self; long enough to be replaced again and again by the 'other'. I am attempting to describe the living, neural processes, each like a mirror which not only reflects the other but *recalls* the other: AS viewing and recalling CS: a reflection recollecting and recognising a reflection in high speed sequence as in a series of stills moving through a projector, and merging into a single image in one place. AS, awareness of 'outside', and CS, aware of an 'outside identity' and its effect on self (Lacan p. 57) become one in a fused perception of self-identity – all feasible because of neurophysiology and time-lapse. And we have a self-generated image of the observing 'I'.

***

There is a richness of internal neurophysiology and of psychodynamic interaction here, both developing over millions of years, if this model or something like it is to be accepted; and, as with the fairground, I am reluctant to leave the cultural setting out of the picture because it is generated by, and generates, the developing, conscious mind. So, as a kind of interval, I will mention the way one of Federico Fellini's greatest films *Eight and a Half* ends, because Fellini was a modern mythologist as well as an artist and entertainer. The film is about childhood, memory, dreams, fantasy, relationships and the frustrations of creative work. Just as the film fades into greyness in a dawn scene of a spaceship on its ramp, everything suddenly comes alive again as hundreds of actors, artists, friends, relatives, designers, poseurs, cameramen, producers, protagonists, antagnoists and God knows who else – the whole credit list presumably – troop down the scaffolding steps arm-in-arm and begin to circle the field. They are led by a small band of musicians (playing the music of Fellini's composer, Nino Roti), and led in turn by a child. And the cameras turn.

***

When self recollects self, one mechanism for animal memory, the other for the memory of a more psychological, cultural world, we have the beginnings of an 'I', and it develops from there, *each self lasting just long enough to register the other, and occurs across myriad neural networks wherever sub-self recognises sub-self as a general, not localised, function of the whole brain.*

Whatever the process, it is continuous and fast: a sense of self is as likely to require a teeming input from inside and outside to maintain it as much as the brain requires a constant flow of oxygenated blood. A chain-reaction would be the wrong metaphor, because that represents a fast-acting expansion based on continuous division. The model proposed is like the toy in the previous illustration (p. 156), but with multiple sub-selves, each based on fleeting incidents and trivialities, occurring faster and faster per moment, until the blur becomes a continuous picture, as in a cinematic film. Here, the shutter (which frames each separate image so that they can be merged into a movie – another achievement of the brain, remember) is being provided by the few milliseconds where the image fades, goes and is replaced by another. The idea is a mirror-image which can see and recall the other mirror-image, which sounds unlikely only if you take the metaphor too literally; but here we are talking about reflections composed of the neural basis for the unconscious, primitive imagery and awareness, and there is no reason to assume there is only one. It is the self-recalling-self which forges what I have called an Io out of these reflections. This is a coarse analogy, and I don't want to take it much further, but it provides a model to meet the need of self being aware of self, and once self is aware of self we have an 'I'.

Could 'slippage' in this system cause phenomena like depersonalisation and *déja vu* (*see* p. 168)?

It would be hard to conceive of human consciousness developing without memory, although there are states of mind where individuals seem aware of themselves as 'I' and able to say 'I have lost my memory' and there are states of mind associated with altered levels of consciousness in which someone may for a time be in a state similar to animal awareness without knowing or perhaps even wondering who or where they are. Memory is usually categorised as short term and long term (*see* Rose 1993), the former being labile and fading in minutes or hours, while some information passes into the long-term memory where it can endure for a lifetime but is not necessarily always accessible. Precisely how memory is stored isn't established, with theories including memory storage in neural circuits or distributed in fields across the cortex. The hippocampus – so called because it looks like a seahorse – is thought to be involved in transfer between short-term and long-term memory, has locomotor connections, and is associated with the limbic system, part of the brain which is particularly involved in mediating and transmitting autonomic and visceral signals – gut feelings; and 'I' involves narrative – literary, historical and autobiographical, not psychology alone.

Memory, like consciousness, has its elusive side: what it is, where it is and how it does what it does. But beyond neuroscience, memory belongs to cultural history too, and Otis (1994), in her book *Organic Memory*, has reviewed a wealth of ways in which the literary and the physical come together, making an analogy between heredity and memory on the one hand with society and the individual on the other which goes well beyond Lamarckism (*see* p. 92). Her account suggests that language and metaphor bridges gaps between our physical and genetic selves, literature and memory in ways consistent, I think, with the account of archetypes given earlier.

None of which quite explains why the Greeks made Mnemosyne, the mother of all the Muses, the goddess of Memory. But it is intriguing that they did, making a mythical connection between memory and creativity. It is another example of what the poets seem to know intuitively and science discusses later. There she is on the cover of this book, astride a seahorse (*Hippocampus erectus*) on a carousel. I chose this picture for the book before I realised fully what it illustrated – I think.

I don't want to take the model any further at this stage, except to say that the 'toy cinema' is a little crude for the extraordinary, complex beauty of what happens. I would prefer a sphere to a carousel (I imagine one made out of many thousands of rapid cycling neural circuits), one that as it turns, following multiple angles of spin, and develops a hologram of the 'I' within it. Also, if the reader will accept the 'cinema' model, it is important not to forget the cultural contributions mentioned earlier, from dreamers and scriptwriters through camera operators and sound engineers, producers, directors, actors, designers, financiers, people who make the tea, people who find hotels for stars, and all the distributors, advertisers, and every kind of myth-maker, including the allotment of roles, and then there are the dreamers in the audience, and what people say about the film publicly and in conversation. These contributions, as I have called them, are from without (culture) but already prepared, archetypally, within, and with individual feelings and perceptions projected out again. All this, meme-like, constitutes the building blocks of the world and consciousness, and it all has its circuitry.

In Figure 9.2 I have tried to rough out a Heath Robinson-type model for the self-conscious, I-generating mind. The distinguished cartoonist's drawings were crazy but if you followed all the levers and ropes and pulleys the things he designed would have worked, after a fashion. My drawing, more cosmic in ambition, doesn't represent even a partially working apparatus, but does include most of the main areas I have been discussing. In the text I have tried to include rough translations between one subject and the ones with which I think connections need to be made. But the move from rough interpretation to finer-tuned communication and then to a common language, if conceivable, has yet to be achieved.

***

Where does a cycle like this begin? That might be an anthromorphic and ultimately illusory question. As touched upon in the last chapter, is it possible that potential and immutable laws of the universe be brought into existence at the moment matter and energy happens, with nothing describable as 'time' beforehand? To the extent that human intuition, spirituality and mythology might be an intellectual guide, mystical Judaism's *Zohar*, so very respectful about Creation, has room for the commentary that before Creation even God may have been potential, not actual. Meanwhile, where are the cultural conceptions that do not yet exist? In Figure 2.2, p. 31?

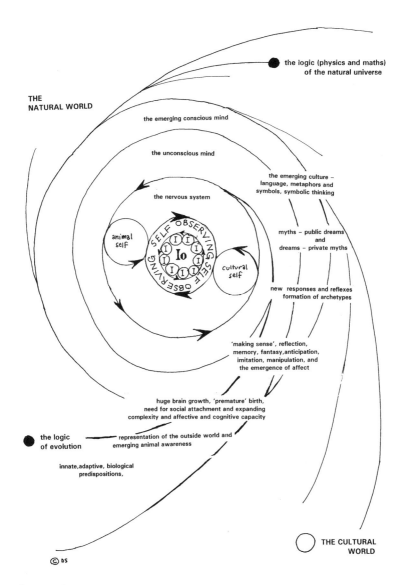

Figure 9.2

Clinical consciousness: a few notes

Messages for psychiatry?

This chapter is not a plea for 'consciousness studies' in healthcare training, still less as another branch of psychiatry. Instead it summarises a few thoughts about clinical practice in psychiatry and related mental health fields which occurred to me while completing the previous primarily theoretical and conceptual chapters.

Consciousness in the textbooks

In its almost 2500 pages, the estimable and monumental *Oxford Textbook of Psychiatry* (Gelder *et al.* 2000) has only one dedicated to disorders of consciousness, though its authors (Sims *et al.* 2000) succeed in covering an impressive range of conditions under this heading; though even then they are primarily those disorders traditionally placed in this category, for example varying states of awareness, disorientation for time, place and person, narrowing of consciousness in delusional states and clouding of consciousness. Disorders of self and body image and depersonalisation (an important and little understood disturbance in the sense of familiarity) are discussed elsewhere, and in Simeon and Abugel (2006) a new key work. Incidentally I am indebted to Sims and his colleagues for two quotations about consciousness: Karl Jaspers' description (1913, in Sims *et al.* 2000) as 'the whole of present mental life' on the one hand, and Lipowski's on the other (1990), that 'the concept of consciousness is wholly redundant'. I suspect that by this Lipowski means that we may simply take consciousness for granted and get on with the job. However, in trying to comprehend the length, breadth and depth of mental life in all its order and disorder, I suggest that our relevant schools of thought are still in their infancy, and we should no more take consciousness for granted than do the physicists, who currently regard it as one of the most enduring of mysteries.

As said, it is not my intention to propose a new hybrid called 'consciousness studies', which would be both tiresome and unnecessary but to see whether the broad notion of consciousness might represent a pragmatic improvement on the clinically traditional 'mental state examination'.

Disorders of consciousness?

Nunn (1997), in a paper entitled 'Diseases of consciousness', touches on a particularly difficult area of the clinical versus social debate, suggesting that this category should include conditions like some allergic disorders, myalgic encephalomyelitis (ME) and anorexia nervosa, because of what he identifies as their significant psychological and socio-cultural elements. However, well-intentioned clinicians often fall out of the frying pan and into the fire here, even attracting hate mail and worse, for by trying to say that some disorders (I hardly dare identify which) have psychological and cultural components, they are accused of denying their reality. Thus, in cultural and in a general sense political terms, the wheel goes full circle and the doctor, once too 'organic', now gets castigated for suggesting that a particular condition may not be 100% physical. This seems like a broadly cultural phenomenon rather than a narrow professional one; and yet it is clear that the proposition that a clinical problem has a psychological facet can in some hands be used (and received) as much as an insult or punishment as an understanding and compassionate viewpoint. There is in this kind of area a long way to go.

Clinical practice and 'mental life'

Nunn's paper and Jaspers' delineation of consciousness as 'the whole of mental life' made me wonder whether the areas I have been discussing as the building blocks of consciousness – not only neurophysiology and psychology but arts, ethics and philosophical positions – would help us in beginning to look at the question of where clinical medicine (I refer particularly to psychiatry and to psychiatric and social aspects of general practice and the workload of casualty departments) tails off and social and educational help begins. That at present this is a fudged area containing overlaps and gaps and many competing views about technical and personal authority is not merely untidy, but results in referral systems which seem to me largely arbitrary, notably in the child psychiatry, psychology and care fields (Steinberg 1983). The healthcare service seems never to satisfy anyone for long, however many personnel it has and however much money is directed into it, and if this is dismissed as mere grumbling one must point to the serious gaps which make the headlines when, for example, whole populations in the UK have no health-service dentists or drugs are allotted on the basis of where people happen to live, and also to the actual cost (billions) in litigation, enquiries and suspended staff and the hidden cost of 'defensive medicine'. This problem will not go away, indeed can only escalate, especially as, to their credit, energetic and ambitious academic departments continually develop new techniques, and, in some cases less to their credit, individuals and the media identify new conditions to worry about. There is no obvious or democratic way we are going to stop new disorders, new treatments and new resources being sought and in this respect healthcare services are on a collision course with reality (Steinberg 2005). My modest proposal, and I do mean modest, considering the scale of the problem, is that if the previous chapters opened up new ideas about what constitutes, in Jaspers' sense, the 'whole of present mental life', applying the broad psychoneurological-cultural framework might go a little way towards delineating mental state disorders from problems in living, or indeed in simply being alive – by which I mean self-management (and child upbringing) by the former and, rather vaguely, a spirituality which is not necessarily religious in any formal sense by the latter. I will mention here, not as a recommendation but for interest, that Freud once suggested that psychoanalysts could represent a new and coming priesthood.

Distinguishing the whole of mental life from mental state systems and disorders – or whole consciousness and its constituents from mental disorder – could be a feasible and useful exercise. An analogy: if I take my car to the garage for a repair I don't want advice on places to go and routes, but someone familiar with all the wires and other gadgetry. If I go to a travel agent about touring somewhere I need quite different advice. This may seem too crude an analogy for clinical practice but, as said, sooner or later choices will have to be made in this area. I can imagine criticism of this suggestion including its encouragement of the much grumbled about 'medical model'. I have argued elsewhere (Steinberg 2005; Tyrer and Steinberg 2005) that simple observation of what actually goes on in medicine shows this is less an entirely organic model of care than an arrangement where A assesses B, makes a diagnosis and prescribes treatment strategy C. This represents the much-criticised 'medical model' no less when undertaken, as it regularly is, by the many psychologists and psychotherapists whose work is equally guided by what they claim to see in their clientele which their clientele cannot. There is an alternative, which I describe below under the general rubric of 'consultative work' in a wider sense than clinical consultation, and which, just possibly, could be a strategy for dealing with wider aspects of consciousness – 'the whole of present mental life' – than with mental states.

If there was some agreement, eventually, about the theoretical basis for whole-life psychology (instead of just the wiring) this could begin to make sense of two important and I think under-researched areas – complementary or alternative medicine and the surprising phenomenon of the placebo.

'Nidotherapy' is a new 'whole of life' approach described by Peter Tyrer and his colleagues at Imperial College in London (Tyrer 2002; Tyrer and Bajaj 2005). It is a development of social approaches to psychiatric care and refers to detailed, collaborative attempts to change the environment rather than the patient. The word derives from *nidus*, Latin for nest, which is a creative environment adapted to fit the creatures that use it, mentioned on earlier pages as part of the cycle by which a brain builds an environment which in turn nutures the mind. If nidotherapy achieves successes, it will be interesting to see how much the newly generated environment, initially 'holding' the patient, in due course effects beneficial change too. For many years, incidentally, I assumed 'therapy' invariably meant 'treatment' with all its clinical implications, until a Greek colleage pointed out that the word comes from *therapeia*, meaning to be of service. One service of nidotherapy may be to minimise 'patient status'.

Consultative work as a strategy for dealing with 'whole life'

I have referred to consultative work and had better explain what it means. Essentially, you could divide 'helping' work as that which is done for you by an expert, and that where the expert's expertise is in helping you sort it out for yourself, the idea being that you learn new skills in the process. In saying this I am well aware that, first, the word 'consultation' is used in all sorts of other ways; and, second, that the idea of teams of consultants charging large fees to organisations and governments for doing what many think they ought to be able to do with their own experts has become somewhat overextended and perhaps tarnished in recent years.

My own concept of consultative work is derived from what seems to help in health and care services, particularly with young people, where the consultant tries to help problem-solving (and clientele) stay with the consultee, to reduce re-referral, reduce the number of new people involved, help the consultee do more than he or she perhaps thought they could, and, if possible, prevent the client (e.g. the pupil of a teacher) becoming the patient of a clinician unless that seems necessary. In consultation nothing is off-limits if the consultee wants to raise it: people's personal ethics, their spirituality, their places of work and employment conditions and resources, even their (and their supervisors') motivation and energy and their possible need for more or special training or even – from elsewhere – counselling; occasionally occupational counselling; anything comes into consultative work's wide net if the consultee thinks it relevant to the issue brought for consultation (Steinberg 1989, 2005). It is particularly relevant in child and adolescent care and therapy, where referrals are quite arbitrary, diagnostic categories uncertain, the 'best' approach often controversial, ethical and legal issues highly complex, and authority and responsibility dispersed between different people (parents and professionals) and agencies. In such all-grey areas consultative approaches can effectively clarify who wants what and who has both the information and the authority to do something. Conceivably, it could contain something useful for other fields too (Steinberg 2004b).

Consultation in this sense is a strategy for 'pure' problem-clarifying and problem-solving without prior assumptions shaping the direction of the interview, and the relative status of those taking part may be described as a joint exploration of what is wanted, what is needed and what is possible (Steinberg 1989, 1992, 2005), an approach which is quite versatile, for example it can be employed in the way we write clinical letters (Steinberg 2000). The essence is that the specialist (e.g. the clinician) brings his or her knowledge and consultative skills to the situation, and the patient or client brings theirs. It casts a wide net, but the more skilled the consultation the more quickly work becomes focused on the three main questions just identified; and, crucially important, the consultant learns from the consultee, as well as vice versa. At its best, it is a problem-focused *educational* approach in which both sides learn, and, if it works, enables consultant as well as consultee to go away more able to handle similar and equivalent matters in the future, and thus there is a fallout in terms of self-help and public education.

However, just as I emphasised that I am not promoting 'consciousness studies' as a panacea, or even a good idea, I am not suggesting that everyone should start using all the technical strategies of consultation. Rather, the broadly consultative, exploratory rather than advisory approach could become a culturally accepted alternative to the didactic, persuasive and prescriptive style of managing each other currently dominating our healthcare culture and politics, left, right and centre. Starting from there, anything possible becomes possible; which is not a mere play on words, because at the moment – and I am thinking of the clinical field – all sorts of perfectly feasible approaches seem opened up by consultative collaboration between professionals, and professionals and their patients (Steinberg 1992, 2005) but appear, mysteriously, to be institutionally beyond reach and not admissible in many academic areas nor as common sense.

Health education and self-help

What we know about the prevention of diseases and the promotion of health needs to be publicised, if it can be done in a balanced kind of way, but this does seem problematic. There will always be headlines announcing 'scientists say' for every twist and turn of the eternal debate about what is or isn't good for us, and as to the state regulating the details of what we do, it would be better if common sense about health became something taught in schools preferably within an academic subject where what's taught should be open to discussion and debate, rather than pressed onto pupils and students by State health and social work enforcers. If there were to be a real cultural shift, a genuine change in the accepted paradigm of what is 'illness' and the responsibility of health professionals, and what is part of life in general, a start could be made in the education of children.

The core subject would be located between human biology, anthropology, and the humanities (in which I would include the classics and the basics of philosophy), and if educationalists respond by saying there can't be any such combined teaching I would say *that* seems to be the trouble. I believe quite young pupils could be taught the beginning of philosophy and how to handle new ideas, especially across the traditional boundaries, with open minds, with a reasonable degree of constructive criticism, within which the scepticism of young people should be encouraged. I would include in my own prescription the origins and meanings of words (like 'illness'), how they are used in literature and poetry – and grammar. Particular attention could be paid to the artificial gaps between different subjects – like art and science – how that came about and how to make connections between them.

But all this would set several cats among the pigeons, especially as, at least in the UK in State schools, and perhaps in some academic areas of the United States, there seems to be an entrenched, institutionalised assumption of the 'correct view' about what should be taught, not taught and how, which is not only conservative to the point of being quite reactionary but which deals with dissidents by accusing them of being 'neo-conservative' or worse. Even to mention political correctness (PC) other than as a self-deprecating joke is seriously non-PC – the ultimate thought crime. It may take the best of science – I mean from the best of scientists who are genuinely open minded, questioning and curious – to counterbalance the politically correct inflexibility of the old guard. In a sense it requires learning about how to learn, which seems to be disappearing from modern curricula. Meanwhile such things are not taught in the healthcare fields, let alone in schools. However, we are as on course for Furedi's or Fitzpatrick's versions of the Therapeutic Society (Fitzpatrick 2000; Furedi 2004), tightly controlled by well-meaning social engineers, as the *Titanic* was for its iceberg, and if we are to divert from that infinitely expensive and ultimately counterproductive goal we should begin now to reverse engines from the over-managed Technological Society and take a wider look at what, and what else, makes us fully human.

In whose own image?

Self, nature, supernature and belief

Are the missing links clear? Attachment theory links the necessities of evolution with an emerging, primal culture. Archetypal theory connects the emerging primal culture with biologically driven dynamic psychology. Dynamic psychology connects the animal mind with cultural identity. The animal mind, much of it behaviour and low-key awareness, plus emerging cultural identity form two kinds of proto-self. When proto-self meets proto-self neurophysiologically, we have the beginnings of 'I' – the self. All this is a continuing, present process – in the culture and in the memory. But remember that all memories are *now*.

***

> *But there is this difference between the record of the rocks and the secrets which are hidden in language: whereas the former can only give us a knowledge of outward, dead things such as forgotten seas and the bodily shapes of prehistoric animals and primitive men, language has preserved for us the inner, living history of man's soul. It reveals the evolution of consciousness. (Owen Barfield, etymologist, 1926)*

To what extent was Barfield overstating the case? Not that much, I think, especially if we may stretch the concept of words, as I have suggested throughout this book, to include all that is symbolic, signifying and metaphoric in culture. The main thesis of this book – there is an attempt at an schematic diagram for it (Figure 9.2) at the end of Chapter 9, albeit something of a firework display – is that while nature provided us with unselfconscious, unknowing awareness, which evolved out of relatively simple representations of the outside world, our cultural environment and relationships provided the possibility of identity; and that when animal awareness and socio-cultural identity meet in the flux of the neuronal networks of the brain, there is a kind of mutual recognition, out of which the observing I, which I have called Io, emerges as a real illusion. It is a meeting of minds, through metaphor.

That is the basis of it, but this miraculous chemistry doesn't happen without the catalysts of memory, fantasy and anticipation, fed by, first, feelings from the individual unconscious mind and, second, with predispositions for imagery from the collective unconscious mind, universal to all people. This requires cultural symbols and relationships, and the memories, fantasies, anticipation, feelings and images *about* cultural symbols and relationships.

I cannot imagine all this without words. The question is sometimes put, often in an either–or way, whether we need words to think with or does thinking generate words? On page 42 I suggested that words are parachuted into the brain with meanings, implicit and explicit, attached; but it can work both ways, in that inchoate feelings and fantasies can find their expression in more and more appropriate symbols until we find the right word for them. Either way, words and their symbolic attachments make memories, fantasies and anticipations possible.

***

In the 1960s on a grainy black-and-white TV screen I watched Don Cupitt, theologian, debating religion with AJ Ayer, logical positivist. Cupitt expounded the case for religion while AJ Ayer, amused and impatient, shook his head. 'No, no, no, no', he was protesting, (or possibly 'yes, yes, yes, yes', because he was agreeing with Cupitt), 'but what you are describing is humanism, not theology'.

Don Cupitt's conclusion in his book *Creation Out of Nothing* (1990) is that God exists in language, first as an audible God of speech, then as the God of writing, and then – now – as the God of language 'as a symbol of where words come from'. You must read Cupitt's argument to see that this is not a simplistic argument. He describes God being seen from classical antiquity 'as a self-founding Creator-Subject who generates both reality and his own knowledge of it, and the human self was regarded as having been made by God in his own image'; later, there was the 'corrective' of the return of the self into nature and into history; and then, with the modern philosophers, Cupitt saw the natural notion of self being challenged by:

> *religion as a way in which the conscious self relates itself to the*
> *upsurging flow of language-and-life-energy that is continuously*

producing and dispersing it. A spirituality that becomes a religious
stance by which we ... cope with our own ephemerality. (Cupitt, 1990)

Cupitt also makes the interesting point that life is a world of language
and meanings within which intelligible action becomes possible, and
only then, *after all this is in place*, can science get going. In words
reminiscent of the anthropic principle (*see* p. 96). Cupitt argues that
'the very large and slightly absurd object that physicists call the
Universe can only be produced if the life-world is already first given'.
(Cupitt, 1990)

***

The most remarkable operation of consciousness is how the mind
makes things matter. This is too easily taken to be just another given.
Perhaps it is thrown off in that fast-spinning reciprocity between the
animal sense of survival and a culturally-indiced narcissism, yet the
subjective feeling that anything at all matters is surely fundamental to
all human motivation.

***

Which else came first, the chicken or the egg? Logically, and
biologically, the egg, naturally, because that was the beginning of
the first creature called a chicken. Whatever laid the egg was something else, albeit a chicken ancestor, some kind of proto-chicken.

By the same token I am curious about the first human face, in all its
expressiveness, intense gaze and beaming response to its mother's
face. This must surely have been extraordinary to the parents who had
never seen this facial mobility. We think it attractive. Would they
have? It might have been grotesque rather than beguiling. It is
possible that changes from the relatively inexpressive, static face of
the ancestors to the extraordinary liveliness of the face of the human
infant developed very gradually over generations, involving small
changes in the neurology and musculature, so that the parent would
not have been too shaken. But it is as least as likely that there was a
watershed, a small change that suddenly made all the difference in
one baby of one mother. Animals are vigilant for infants that don't fit
the bill, and may neglect or kill them. It is likely that the attachment
dynamic before and after the appearance of the first baby like this
would have been different. Which came first? The bizarre new infant

or the unconditionally loving mother? Are there any myths that echo such a change?

***

In a talk on the God-Deity in the Brain at a conference on Art and Mind, Professor Todd Murphy of the Laurentian University, Canada, affirmed his experience of the power of prayer *and* his assumption that there was no external God. He asked, with due humility and puzzlement: 'then who am I praying to? Myself? Is God in the Mind? Would that diminish the concept of a Divinity? Why? (Murphy, 2005). It may seem a revolutionary notion to some, though in Islam I understand it has been said 'God is closer than the jugular'. Why project notions of God away, first onto mountains, then onto clouds, then into the sky and finally out into space? Is it something to do with Man's vision narrowing as his known world expands? Is it a kind of banishment? Or is it to maintain a mystery, perhaps to maintain the control of the projector, or to perpetuate a state of non-knowing?

My own act of faith, if that is the right word for it, is in the vast potential of the human mind, most of which I suspect is as yet untapped. The kind of mind I have been describing has untapped depths, whether these are imagined neuropsychologically as layer after layer of the unconscious mind, fluid and dynamic as the oceans, or culturally, in terms of imagination and language, where words, symbols and the imagination may take the conscious mind into new, i.e. newly minted, territory. The 'grappling iron' again (or track-laying vehicle), throwing out a word for an unclear thought, then advancing with its help.

But there is a shared, communal world outside too, of all those words, concepts, tales, things which I swept up together as the arts; this is as unlimited as the unconscious mind; remember all those billions upon billions of possible neural connections on the one hand, and all those words that could be made out of my five by five alphabetical grid on the other. Add to this 'sandwich' of the unknown and perhaps as-yet-unknowable both within and without, plus the physical limitations of our senses of sight, sound, taste, smell and feeling, and what fills the sandwich – a slice of consciousness – seems very thin indeed. In general, the human race thinks it's pretty good, on balance, and with good reason. But if the above outline of what's outside the sandwich is even on the way to the truth, then comparatively speaking we know next to nothing.

Precognition, for example. Seeing the future isn't possible, because by definition the future hasn't happened yet. But to what extent could an active, busy brain, using more of its memory and more of its scanning capacity than the tiny part we usually employ, predict from millions of signals *probabilities* about situations and people? Quite a lot of folklore has been quite reliable about animal and even plant activity predicting events to do with warmth, water and food. Could we do even better? At what point does prediction differ from precognition? (*See* Monod, 1972).

Fanciful it may seem, but computerised 'data mining', predicting from millions of bits of information on a situation about a future one, is now well within the capacity of computers, and the unfettered brain is mightier than the computer. Data-processing CCTV can tell with a reasonable degree of predictability, one that is likely to improve, the likely behaviour of people or groups as they proceed along a street. Experienced head waiters, so it is said, begin to open the very bottle of wine that they know customers are likely to want as soon as they see the body language of the group as they enter the restaurant. You only have to extrapolate from these examples and suddenly the crazy idea of precognition seems feasible, and natural rather than supernatural. Large proportions of populations believe in various forms of paranormal activity and extra-sensory perception (ESP), for which the scientific evidence is scanty if it exists at all. I mention such things not because I believe they exist in forms in which they are commonly believed in, but because with its inbuilt intuition, paranoia and creativity the human race is probably onto something, even if, as yet, it doesn't quite know what it is.

I put it this way because like my primitive and slightly batty proto-human, curious about what was on the other side of the river, and being an optimist (like he or she was) who believes that the human race will still be around for a million years or more, and is only just starting out, I am curious about what is yet to become known. If we can disentangle ideas of the supernatural, and spirituality and divinity from all the pride and the prejudice and the institutionalised belief-systems that distort them and our capacity even for debate, we may find something there somewhere, though no doubt as removed from what we perceive today as, say, a flash of lightning which drove a remote ancestor into a cave with fears of aerial gods or demons is different from today's TV and Internet; or even as what we now know as the Internet will be like within the lifetimes of our grandchildren.

The same physics, the same energy, but different information and understanding.

Where, by the way, is the Internet? If you read accounts of it, for example Gordon Graham's, you will get a convincing description of a new way of being; that 'it is not merely possible to observe the world of the Internet; it is possible to exist and to act in it' (Graham 1999). The Internet, leaving aside the batteries and the wiring, is mostly in the mind.

***

At the start of this book I referred to a change of mind. When starting the book I had challenged the reader, and in a sense myself, to choose between the natural or the supernatural when it came to the origin of the self, on the grounds that the issue couldn't be fudged: we, the whole of us, came from either chemistry or divinity, and I was primarily on the side of the molecules. But are the arts, culture, ideas in general, and the symbols and words in which they are recorded, natural? Is all this stuff, made partly of memory, partly of fantasy, and partly of God knows what in terms of what the unconscious can generate and the culture or microculture provides, really natural, i.e. *material*? But I wouldn't call it supernatural either. Is there a third category where – among other things – the observing I, the self, has its domain? What do we call these abstractions which, in thought as well as fixed on the record like pinned butterflies, continue whether their creators are around or not? 'Non-natural' is a bit dismissive. Para-natural? Internatural? Intranatural? Epinatural?

***

Aldous Huxley, in his classic work (1954) on taking the drug mescalin (precursor to other powerful hallucinogenic agents), speculated that the pharmacology opened up the mind to material on a cosmic scale that, ordinarily, the mind had to screen out to get through the day. Creative people in all fields lift that screen a little, with variable results. If such intuition (or even 'ancient wisdom') is 90% junk and 10% brilliance, what about the brilliance? But, as in Kipling's poem (*see* p. 46), there is a risk of madness here. Scientists get emotional when others act on conviction while they have to limit themselves to painstakingly observing the observable and measuring the measurable. Their approach is essential. But so also is the intuitive, speculative world of artists and philosophers, and the new kind of scientists emerging in quantum physics and cosmology, who – curiously, just like psycho-analysts – explore at the very edges of the universe on the one hand and of consciousness on the other. I suspect the outcome will be a major paradigm shift – over the next few thousand years – one which will shift consciousness to a different kind of plane or place. Not better, nor worse; just different, though perhaps better suited to a different world in which the objective is so under reliable control (I mean housing, feeding, health, energy supply, the ecology) that the human race will be able to afford a less obviously technical, more obviously aesthetic, intuitive and subjective state of consciousness and kind of world. What a renaissance that would be. But at the moment (if we could know them), we would, no doubt, think our descendants mad; just as they would rightly think us mad. If you doubt the latter, look around.

***

Despite Cupitt, it is hard to pin religion and spirituality down. I think both a little mad, like belief, but absolutely necessary, adaptive mad-nesses, and therefore, paradoxically, in one perfectly proper and important context not mad. Both are essential parts of the equipment that has enabled the human race to adapt and survive. The ultimate clarity of ambiguity is also seen in Fellini's quote (1987) from his 'real dreams' (*see* p. 9), or if you ask yourself about war: is military conflict mad, frankly psychotic? Unloading bombs and bullets onto people? Or is it the only logical course for self-defence when politics (what Churchill called jaw jaw, as preferable to war-war) fails? The answer to both questions is, unfortunately for us, yes. Tolerance of ambiguity, like a sense of humour, is often seen as a mark of maturity and civilisation. It holds situations while a temporarily unavoidable moral or practical muddle slowly clarifies.

***

The artist, anthropologist and psychoanalyst Erik Erikson also invoked ambiguity and duality when he distinguished between the human ego and the self, saying that the self should move beyond narcissism to love of the 'I' 'as an experience which conveys some world order and spiritual sense, no matter how dearly it has to be paid for ... it is the acceptance of one's life and life cycle as something that had to be'

(Erikson, 1965). That resolution enables the enduring strength Erikson described as developing renunciation and wisdom and the acceptance of death; the opposite being despair. The essence of the most positive outcome was being able to celebrate *having been*. (Though what can be done if we lose all our memory?) *Being* is an aspect of life and consciousness which is explored more in existential philosophy than in most studies of consciousness. Erikson would have been thinking adaptively when he suggested than if adults did not fear death their children would not fear life. He stated the alternatives needing some resolution by the end of life as ego integrity versus despair. David Taylor reinterpreted the alternatives, starkly and more poetically, as 'We have been' versus 'we have been robbed' (Taylor, 1972). One may consider in this context Richard Dawkins' ambiguously comforting words (*see* p. 39) and Mervyn Peake's thought, 'to have lived at all is miracle enough'. It is from his poem *The Glassblowers* (1950) and is on his headstone, in Burpham, in Sussex (Gilmour, 1970). 'To have been' is rather nice, I think, especially in Latin – *fuisse* – when it sounds like a zephyr, a soft breeze. Inspiration; expiration. Try it.

***

To return to the Preface with which the book started, first, I am less sure now that the universe and its (that is, our) minds can so readily be divided into *either* the product of materialism *or* the creation of a divinity. Mind and its origins and productions are too remarkable, I now think, for so simple a dichotomy. Although I do not think along with Berkeley that the universe is only in the mind, there does seem to be philosophical evidence that the human mind orders our universe by seeing in it the order that suits us. The nervous systems and the minds we have evolved to date, including on the one hand the kinds of metaphors and mathematics at our disposal for shoehorning information into our minds, and on the other the range of archetypes we have evolved, provides us with only one of innumerable possible universes.

The question I am left with is about the status of two kinds of phenomena. First, in the broadest sense, the arts and all that is mental and cultural in our group awareness and in our memories, from any kind of abstractions you care to name, including mathematics, arts, music, philosophies, and beliefs and the way they are not only embedded in our culture, in the very words we use, but in our collectively human archetypal experience. As asked before, is all this stuff, this extraordinary, vast and burgeoning noosphere, natural or 'epinatural'? As a baby appears on the planet, as tuned in as the finest receiver, it starts sucking in all these abstractions, with words, symbols and symbolism as the catalysts, and it may continue like that for a hundred years, producing or refining psychological theories, mathematical equations and the arts as it goes (among other activities) and always questioning, questioning, questioning.

Second, it seems to me that there is something more enduring, that was there even before the Big Bang, but which also is an abstraction and even, in a sense, an illusion; although as we have seen with consciousness, there's nothing wrong (or unreal) about abstractions and delusions. I mean the fundamental laws of the universe –the kind that Penrose talks about (*see* p. 148), and which carry for this mathematical non-initiate a kind of conviction, although speaking for myself I understand them no more than – I imagine – most people who make up the world's religious audiences really grasp theology. Take the latest mystery within physics – gravity – which doesn't fit any of the present quantum rules. Its laws are presumably immutable; but these laws don't appear until the universe appears. Once we have that dual phenomenon, mass and energy – but not before – gravity appears. If the universe completely disappeared I imagine, such is my understanding, gravity would go with it; but would it and all the other physical laws be there as immutable possibilities in a non-existent universe, appearing with the appearance of mass and energy?

But it takes a mind to know a law of gravity when it sees one. Is Mind, and its potential for growing 'I's, neither natural nor supernatural, but similarly inherent in the universe as something that's bound to happen once a nervous system evolves from a protozoan into a complex, good-enough neural network?

Do the laws of language, like those of maths, pre-exist in the universe-to-be, awaiting only a mind and a voice? Could God pre-exist in the universe as a concept involving potential for mathematics, indeed potential for gravity, and potential for language, and grow further into being as mass, then life, and then Consciousness appear? Until a being evolves who – as, in one way or another, many basic and especially mystic religious accounts argue – God and man gaze at each other. Have those who argue for intelligent design allowed for this? Are those who project their own ideas of what is 'intelligent' onto a God being a little presumptuous?

The phrase 'God made Man in his own image' seems ambiguous, and perhaps was meant to be. The Kabbalah, by which I mean the original and scholarly Jewish mysticism, describes the creation of Man as God needing Man in order to see God, and that while the Zohar (the classical kabbalistic text) is an account of a single God, it also indicates *degrees* of God from absolute nothingness (the highest grade) to the lowest, which is the conscious soul of man. It also suggests that there is more than one kind of possible universe. Is this kind of theological yet at the same time psychological and poetic exposition – characteristic of mystical writings for example in Gnosticism, the Zohar and in the mystic forms of the major religions generally (e.g. Happold 1970; Scholem 1961; Underhill 1961; Shah 1968; Hoffman 1981; Matt 1983; Pitchon 1988) – a further example of poetic vision, the kind of grasp of how the world is? Or of divine or intuitive messages? And what is the difference? As we saw, Cupitt (1985, 1990, 1998) in his long and thorough search concludes that God exists in *words*. He asks: what is philosophy, but language; and after all – what's language? And then *'But, what isn't?'*

There is an intriguing consonance between the problems of grasping the outer limits of mind science and our similar problems in comprehending the universe, as shown by a certain amount of uncertainty in quantum physics. Are these different fields of study, the one soft, fuzzy and intuitive and the other hard, mathematical and in parts experimentally provable, arching round to *meet*? To tie a belt around our explorations like a kind of cosmic straitjacket? Kipling's prayer (*see* p. 46) again?

***

If we accept the evolutionary importance of belief, of absolute conviction (*see* p. 34) whatever the evidence, and therefore its role as a natural imperative, we must deal with two opposing theses: (1) that God exists, and is extraordinary; and (2) that God does not exist. They are not all fools, on either side. But suppose (a) a God with all the qualities – give or take a few myths and all the human political and manipulative spin and deception – attributed to God by the more thoughtful theologists does exist; and (b) that God with all these qualities is also in and of the mind, perhaps of all minds as a collective archetype, and none the less astonishing for that. Is that a tenable proposition? If so, what would that say about Mind and about God?

***

The more scientific proponents of intelligent design are trying to explain how on earth such finely tuned creatures as ourselves and our animal cousins could conceivably have developed given (in their view) the limits of the time span and Darwinian mechanisms available. Meyer, for example (2005), reviewing what many others have pointed out before, has argued that the intracellular adaptive mechanisms of many cells (for example bacteria) are not merely complex but numerous, and a proportion would have to be in place before the potentially adaptive end-result, for example flagellar 'rotary engines' enabling the organism's movement and survival. This implies a kind of inbuilt foresight, because without what seems to be an end-result actually in place from the start, the preceding steps would not have survived. In other words, several of the mutually-dependent parts all need to be there at the same time, rather than proceeding one by one and stepwise as in the Darwinian model. It appears that there is more than enough information in the cell (in DNA and RNA) to allow for this extraordinary evolution but as Meyer says it 'defies explanation by the forces of chemical necessity'. And then there are the mini-nervous systems in the microtubules of single cells, postulated by Penrose (2006) and others and powered by a version of gravity. Could they conceivably drive aspects of chemical and cellular life in an local adaptive direction that, neural-like and fractal-like, is repeated at higher levels of organisation? Recent work suggests that even amoebae may 'sleep' (Horne 2006). (Do they dream?)

Earlier I suggested that there are two possible answers to the bafflement of intelligent design's proponents; one is that the several thousand million years of life on earth is far longer than we are really able to imagine. The other is that the anthropic principle (*see* pp. 96–7) explains it, by our having the kinds of minds that neatly fit the world we know, so we assume that it is the best of all possible worlds, and our minds the best of all possible minds. In other words, a kind of delusional fixed conviction.

But back to which came first, universe shaping mind, or mind shaping universe, or whether God first gazed upon Man, or Man first gazed upon God, or who made whom in whose image. We may even believe that ultimately there are reciprocities here, cycles, and that nagging away at 'yes, but how did the cycle *start*?' might be a flaw in our reasoning. Perhaps cyclical causation is an immutable law too.

But still, even then, what if

References

Aitchison J (1989) *The Articulate Mammal: an introduction to psycholinguistics.* Routledge, London.

Aitchison J (1996) *The Seeds of Speech.* Cambridge University Press, Cambridge.

Arnheim R (1966) *Towards a Psychology of Art.* Faber and Faber, London.

Arnheim R (1992) *To the Rescue of Art: essays.* University of California Press, California.

Augustine St (1961) *Confessions.* R Pine-Coffin (ed. and trans.). Penguin, London.

Bachelard G (1964) *The Poetics of Space.* Orion, New York.

Bahn P (2005) Cradle of thought. Paper presented at Art and Mind Conference: Religion, Art and the Brain (10–13 March), Winchester, Hampshire.

Barfield O (1926) In: *History in English Words.* Faber, London.

Barkow J, Cosmides L and Tooby J (1992) *The Adapted Mind. Evolutionary psychology and the generation of culture.* Oxford University Press, Oxford.

Baron-Cohen S (2003) *The Essential Difference.* Allen Lane, London.

Barrow J (1995) *The Artful Universe.* Clarendon Press, Oxford.

Barrow J and Tipler F (1986) *The Anthropic Cosmological Principle.* Clarendon Press, Oxford.

Barthes R (1973) *Mythologies.* Paladin, London.

Barthes R (1977) *Image, Music, Text.* Fontana, London.

Bateson G (1973) *Steps to an Ecology of Mind.* Paladin, St Albans.

Bateson G (1979) *Mind and Nature: a necessary unity.* Wildwood House, London.

Benvenuto B and Kennedy R (1986) *The Works of Jacques Lacan: an introduction.* Free Association Books, London.

Berger P and Luckman T (1967) *The Social Construction of Reality.* Penguin, London.

Berleant A (2004) The aesthetics of art and nature. In: A Carlson and A Berleant (eds) *The Aesthetics of Natural Environments.* Chapter 3. Broadview Press, Ontario.

Birdwhistell R (1970) *Kinesics and Context.* Pennsylvania University Press, Philadelphia.

Blackmore S (1999) *The Meme Machine.* Oxford University Press, Oxford.

Blackmore S (2002) Meme machines and consciousness. In: R Carter (ed.) *Consciousness.* Weitenfeld and Nicolson, London. pp. 241–3.

Block N, Flanagan O and Güzeldere G (eds) (1998) *The Nature of Consciousness: philosophical debates.* MIT Press, Cambridge, MA, and London.

Bloom H (2002) *Genius.* Fourth Estate, London.

Bohm D (1974) On the subjectivity and objectivity of knowledge. In: J Lewis (ed.) *Beyond Chance and Necessity.* Garnstone Press, London.

Bohm D (1980) *Wholeness and the Implicate Order.* Routledge and Kegan Paul, London.

Bohr N (1963) Causality and complementarity. In: *Atomic Physics and Human Knowledge. Essays 1958–1962, Vol III*. Oxbow Press, Woodbridge, CT.

Bolton D and Hill J (1996) *Mind, Meaning and Mental Disorder*. Oxford University Press, Oxford.

Booker C (2004) *The Seven Basic Plots*. Continuum, London.

Boorstin D (2001) *The Creators*. Phoenix, London.

Bowlby J (1969) *Attachment and Loss: Volume 1. Attachment*. The Hogarth Press, London.

Bowlby J (1973) *Attachment and Loss: Volume 2. Separation: anxiety and anger*. The Hogarth Press, London.

Bowlby J (1979) *Attachment and Loss: Volume 3. Loss*. Tavistock, London.

Brand-Claussen B, Jadi I and Douglas C (1997) *Beyond Reason: art and psychosis*. Hayward Gallery, London.

Brandon R (1999) *Surreal Lives. The Surrealists 1917–1945*. Macmillan, London.

Breton A (1969) *Conversations: the autobiography of surrealism*. M Polizzotti (trans.). Gallimard, Paris (1969); Marlowe, New York (1993).

Brooke R (1991) *Jung and Phenomenology*. Routledge, London.

Brown JAC (1961) *Freud and the Post-Freudians*. Penguin, London.

Browning R (1855) *Andrea del Sarto*. Smith and Elder, London.

Bullen J (1994) Hardy's *The Wellbeloved*, sex and theories of germ plasm. In: P Mallet and R Draper (eds) *A Spacious Vision: essays on Hardy*. The Patten Press, Newmill.

Burnshaw S (1982) *The Seamless Web*. George Braziller, New York.

Campbell J (1974) *The Masks of God. Volume 4: creative mythology*. Viking, London.

Cardinal R (1972) *Outsider Art*. Praeger Publishers, New York.

Carter R (2002) *Consciousness*. Weidenfeld and Nicolson, London.

Chalmers D (1996) *The Conscious Mind*. Oxford University Press, Oxford.

Chomsky N (1971) *Chomsky; selected readings*. J Allen and P van Buren (eds). Oxford University Press, Oxford.

Clocksin W (1995) Knowledge, representation and myth. In: J Cornwell (ed.) *Nature's Imagination*. Chapter 12. Oxford University Press, Oxford.

Collins C (1994) *The Vision of the Fool and Other Writings*. Golgonooza Press, Ipswich.

Collins J (1989) *Cecil Collins*. Tate Gallery, London.

Cooramaswamy A (1950) In: E Gill (ed.) *The Transformation of Nature in Art*. Devin Adair, New York.

Crick F (1994) *The Astonishing Hypothesis*. Simon and Schuster Ltd, London.

Cupitt D (1985) *The Sea of Faith*. BBC Publications, London.

Cupitt D (1990) *Creation Out of Nothing*. SCM Press, London.

Cupitt D (1998) *After God*. Phoenix, London.

Damasio A (2000) *The Feeling of What Happens*. William Heinemann, London.

Davies P (1982) *The Accidental Universe*. Cambridge University Press, Cambridge.

Davies P (1992) *The Mind of God*. Simon and Schuster, London.

Davies P and Brown J (1986) *The Ghost in the Atom*. Cambridge University Press, Cambridge.

Dawkins R (1976) *The Selfish Gene*. Oxford University Press, Oxford.

Dawkins R (1982) *The Extended Phenotype*. Oxford University Press, Oxford.

Dawkins R (1998) *Unweaving the Rainbow*. Allen Lane, The Penguin Press, London.

Dennett D (1969) *Content and Consciousness*. Routledge and Kegan Paul, London.

Dennett D (1990) Memes and the exploitation of imagination. *Journal of Aesthetics and Art Criticism*. **48**: 127–35.

Dennett D (1991) *Consciousness Explained*. Allen Lane, The Penguin Press, London.

Dennett D (1997) *Kinds of Minds*. Weidenfeld and Nicolson, London.

Dubuffet J (1967) In: *Notes for the Well-lettered (Prospectus et tous écrits suivants)*. Quoted in Thevoz, 1976.

Dunne J (1958) *An Experiment with Time*. Faber and Faber, London.

Edelman G (1987) *Neural Darwinism*. Basic Books, New York.

Edelman G (1989) *The Remembered Present*. Basic Books, New York.

Edelman G (1992) *Bright Air, Brilliant Fire*. Basic Books, New York.

Edelman G (1995) Memory and the individual soul. In: J Cornwell (ed.) *Nature's Imagination*. Chapter 13. Oxford University Press, Oxford.

Edelman G (2005) *Wider Than the Sky*. Penguin, London.

Ehrenzweig A (1965) *The Psycho-Analysis of Artistic Vision and Hearing*. George Braziller, New York.

Erikson E (1965) *Childhood and Society*. Hogarth, London.

Evans P (1972) Henri Ey's concepts of the organisation of consciousness and its disorganisation: an extension of Jacksonian theory. *Brain*. **95**(2): 413–20.

Fellini F (1987) Real dreams. *Omnibus*. BBC TV.

Fine P (1979) Lamarckian ironies in contemporary biology. *Lancet*. **2 June (i)**: 1181–2.

Fineberg J (2000) *Art Since 1940: strategies of being*. Laurence King, London.

Fitzpatrick M (2000) *The Tyranny of Health*. Brunner Routledge, London.

Forster EM (1910) *Howard's End*. Penguin Books, London (1989).

Foucault M (1967) *Madness and Civilisation*. Tavistock, London.

Fowles J (1984) Introduction to J Fowles and J Draper, *Thomas Hardy's England*. Jonathan Cape, London.

Frawley W (1997) *Vygotsky and Cognitive Science*. Harvard University Press, London.

Freud S (1927) The structure of the psyche. In: J Strachey (trans.) (1981) *Collected Works*. Standard edition. Hogarth, London.

Freud S (1950) *Totem and Taboo*. Routledge and Kegan Paul, London.

Freud S (1952) *Introductory Lectures on Psychoanalysis*. George Allen and Unwin, London.

Freud S (1954) *The Interpretation of Dreams*. J Strachey (trans.). George Allen and Unwin, London.

Freud S (1959) *Two Short Accounts of Psychoanalysis*. Penguin, London.

Furedi F (2004) *Therapy Culture. Cultivating vulnerability in an uncertain age*. Routledge, London.

Gane M (1991) *Baudrillard: critical and fatal theory*. Routledge, London.

Gazzaniga M (1994) *Nature's Mind*. Penguin, London.

Gelder M, Lopez-Ibor J and Andreasen N (2000) *New Oxford Textbook of Psychiatry*. Oxford University Press, Oxford.

Genet J (1957) *The Balcony*. Faber and Faber, London.

Gilbert P (1992) *Depression: the evolution of powerlessness*. Laurence Erlbaum, Hillsdale, NJ.

Gilmour M (1970) *A World Away: a memoir of Mervyn Peake*. Victor Gollancz, London.

Gladwell M (2002) *The Tipping Point*. Abacus, London.

Glyn-Jones A (1996) *Holding Up a Mirror*. Century, London.

Goethe JW (1832) *Faust*. In: A Hayward (trans.) (1908). Hutchinson and Co., London.

Golding W (1955) *The Inheritors*. Faber and Faber, London.

Goldman A (1998) Consciousness, folk psychology and cognitive science. In: N Block, O Flanagan and G Güzeldere (eds) *The Nature of Consciousness*. Chapter 5. MIT Press, Cambridge, MA, and London.

Goonatilake S (1991) The neural system and phenotypal information. In: S Goonatilake (ed.) *The Evolution of Information: lineages in gene, culture and artefact*. Chapter 3. Pinter, New York.

Gould SJ (1989) *Wonderful Life*. Hutchinson Radius, London.

Graham G (1999) *The Internet. A philosophical enquiry*. Routledge, London.

Greenfield S (1997) *The Human Brain. A guided tour*. Weidenfeld and Nicolson, London.

Greenfield S (1998) *The Private Life of the Brain*. Allen Lane, London.

Gregory R (1970) *The Intelligent Eye*. Weidenfeld and Nicolson, London.

Gregory R (1987) The unconscious. In: R Gregory (ed.) *The Oxford Companion to the Mind*. Oxford University Press, Oxford.

Gregory R (1997) *Mirrors in Mind*. Penguin, London.

Gregory R (2005) Virtual realities of the mind. Paper presented at Art and Mind Conference: Religion, Art and the Brain (10–13 March), Winchester, Hampshire, UK.

Güzeldere G (1998) The many faces of consciousness: a field guide. In: N Block, O Flanagan and G Güzeldere (eds) *The Nature of Consciousness*. MIT Press, Cambridge, MA, and London.

Happold F (1970) *Mysticism*. Penguin, London.

Hardy B (2000) *Thomas Hardy. Imagining imagination*. Athlone Press, London.

Hardy T (1897) *The Pursuit of the Well-Beloved: a sketch of a temperament*. Macmillan, London.

Hayward J (ed.) (1929) *John Donne. Complete poetry and selected prose*. The Nonesuch Press, London.

Heidegger M (1959) *An Introduction to Metaphysics*. R Manheim (trans.). Yale University Press, New Haven.

Heil J (1998) *Philosophy of Mind*. Routledge, London.

Hepburn J (2004) Landscape and the metaphysical imagination. In: A Carlson and A Berleant (eds) *The Aesthetics of Natural Environments*. Chapter 6. Broadview Press, Ontario.

Hinshelwood RD (1994) *Clinical Klein*. Free Association Books, London.

Hoffman E (1981) *The Way of Splendor: Jewish mysticism and modern psychology*. Shambhalah, London.

Hofstadter D (1979) *Godel, Eicher, Bach. An eternal golden braid*. Basic Books, New York.

Hofstadter D and Dennett D (1981) *The Mind's I*. Basic Books, New York.

Holmes J (1993) *John Bowlby and Attachment Theory*. Routledge, London.

Horne J (2006) *Sleepfaring*. Oxford University Press, Oxford.

Horrobin D (2001) *The Madness of Adam and Eve: how schizophrenia shaped humanity*. Bantam, London.

Humphrey N (1984) *Consciousness Regained*. Oxford University Press, Oxford.

Humphrey N (1995) *Soul Searching: human nature and supernatural belief.* Chatto and Windus, London.

Humphrey N (2002) *The Mind Made Flesh*. Oxford University Press, Oxford.

Huxley A (1954) *The Doors of Perception*. Chatto and Windus, London.

Jacobi J (1968) *The Psychology of CG Jung*. Routledge and Kegan Paul, London.

Jacobi J (1971) Complex/archetype/symbol. In: *The Work of CG Jung*. Bollingen Series LV11. Princeton University Press, New York.

Jaspers K (1913) *General Psychopathology*. Springer, Heidelberg.

Jaynes J (1976) *The Origin of Consciousness in the Breakdown of the Bicameral Mind*. Houghton Mifflin, Boston.

Johnson M (1987) *The Body in the Mind*. University of Chicago, Chicago.

Johnson M and Morton J (1991) *Biology and Cognitive Development: the case of face recognition*. Blackwell, Oxford.

Jung CG (1922) On the relation of analytical psychology to poetry. In: *The Spirit of Man* (1966). *Collected Works*. Routledge and Kegan Paul, London.

Jung CG (1928) On psychic energy. In: *The Structure of Dynamic Aspects of the Psyche* (1954). *Collected Works*. Routledge and Kegan Paul, London.

Jung CG (1954) Archetypes of the collective unconscious. In: *CG Jung Collected Works*. 9(i): 3–41. Routledge and Kegan Paul, London.

Kandinsky W (1946) *On the Spiritual in Art.* Solomon R Guggenheim Foundation, New York.

Keeble B (1994) In: C Collins (ed.) *The Vision of the Fool and Other Writings*. Golgonooza Press, Ipswich.

Kellner D (1995) *Baudrillard: a critical reader*. Blackwell, Oxford.

Kipling R (1922) The prayer of Miriam Cohen. In: R Kipling (ed.) *Rudyard Kipling's Verse 1885–1918: inclusive edition*. Hodder and Stoughton, London.

Kirschner M and Gerhart J (2005) *The Plausibility of Life: resolving Darwin's dilemma.* Yale University Press, Yale.

Knox J (2003) *Archetype, Attachment, Analysis.* Brunner Routledge, London.

Kübler G (1962) *The Shape of Time.* Yale University Press, Yale.

Laing R (1967) The politics of experience. In: *The Politics of Experience and the Bird of Paradise.* Penguin, London.

Langer S (1953) *Feeling and Form.* Routledge and Kegan Paul, London.

Leach E (1976) *Culture and Communication: the logic by which symbols are connected.* Cambridge University Press, Cambridge.

Leader D and Groves G (1995) *Lacan for Beginners.* Icon Books, Cambridge.

LeDoux J (2002) *The Synaptic Self.* Macmillan, London.

Leja M (1993) *Reframing Abstract Expressionism.* Yale University Press, New Haven.

Lem S (1961) *Solaris.* Faber and Faber, London.

Lévi-Strauss C (1967) *Structural Anthropology.* Anchor, Garden City.

Levin D (1985) *The Body's Recollection of Being.* Routledge and Kegan Paul, London.

Lewis-Williams D (2002) *The Mind in the Cave.* Thames and Hudson, London.

Lipowski Z (1990) *Delirium.* Oxford University Press, Oxford.

Lodge D (2002) *Consciousness and the Novel.* Secker and Warburg, London.

London J (1908) *Before Adam.* T Werner Laurie, London.

Lorenz K (1977) *Behind the Mirror.* Methuen, London.

Luria A (1976) Emergence and transition. In: J Pickering and M Skinner (1990) *From Sentience to Symbols.* University of Toronto Press, Toronto.

Lyons J (1988) Origins of language. In: AC Fabian (ed.) *Origins.* Cambridge University Press, Cambridge.

Lyons J (1991) *Chomsky.* Fontana, London

MacLean P (1985) Evolutionary psychiatry and the triune brain. *Psychological Medicine.* **15**: 219–21.

McDowell M (2001) Principles of organisation: a dynamic systems view of the archetype-as-such. *Journal of Analytical Psychology.* **46**(4): 637–54.

Maizels J (1996) *Raw Creation.* Phaidon, London.

Malik K (2000) *Man, Beast and Zombie.* Weidenfeld and Nicolson, London.

Malraux A (1958) Sketch for a psychology of the moving pictures. In: S Langer (ed.) *Reflections on Art.* Galaxy, New York.

Mandelbrot B (1977) *The Fractal Geometry of Nature.* Freeman, New York.

Maritain J (1954) *Creative Intuition in Art and Poetry.* Harvill Press, London.

Matt D (1983) *Zohar. The Book of Enlightenment.* SPCK, London.

McCrone J (1990) *The Ape That Spoke.* Macmillan, London.

Meyer S (ed.) (2005) *Darwinism, Design and Public Education.* State University Press, Michigan.

Miller D (ed.) (1983) *A Pocket Popper.* Fontana, London.

Monod J (1972) *Chance and Necessity.* Collins, London.

Murphy T (2005) *Deity in the Brain?* Paper presented at Art and Mind Conference: Religion, Art and the Brain. (10–13 March), Winchester, Hampshire, UK.

Nunn C (1997) Diseases of consciousness? *Journal of the Royal Society of Medicine.* **90**: 400–1.

Orians G and Heerwagen J (1992) Evolved responses to landscapes. In: J Barkow, L Cosmides and J Tooby (eds) *The Adapted Mind.* Oxford University Press, Oxford.

Otis L (1994) *Organic Memory.* University of Nebraska Press, London.

Pagels H (1982) Schrödinger's cat. In: *The Cosmic Code.* Simon and Schuster, New York.

Paglia C (2001) *Sexual Personae.* Yale Nota Bene, Yale.

Pais A (1991) Niels Bohr's times. In: *Physics, Polity and Philosophy.* Clarendon Press, Oxford.

Parkes C (1969) Separation anxiety: an aspect of the search for a lost object. In: MH Lader (ed.) *Studies of Anxiety.* Royal Medico-Psychological Association, London, and Headley Brothers, Ashford.

Parkes C (1971) Psychosocial transitions: a field for study. *Social Science and Medicine.* **5**: 101–15.

Peake M (1950) To live at all. In: *The Glassblowers.* Eyre and Spottiswoode, London.

Penrose R (1990) *The Emperor's New Mind.* Oxford University Press, Oxford.

Penrose R (1994) *Shadows of the Mind.* Oxford University Press, Oxford.

Penrose R (2004) Essay, consciousness. In: R Gregory (ed.) *Oxford Companion to the Mind* (2e). Oxford University Press, Oxford.

Penrose R (2006) *The Road to Reality.* Vintage, London.

Pine-Coffin E (trans.) (1961) *St Augustine.* Penguin, London.

Pinker S (1994) *The Language Instinct.* Allen Lane, The Penguin Press, London.

Pinker S (1997) *How the Mind Works.* Allen Lane, The Penguin Press, London.

Pitchon E (1988) Models of explanation in kabbalah and psychoanalysis. In: H Cooper (ed.) *Soul Searching: studies in Judaism and psychotherapy.* SCM Press, London.

Polizzotti M (1995) *Revolution of the Mind. The life of André Breton.* Bloomsbury, London.

Popper K (1999) *Unended Quest.* Routledge, London.

Popper K and Eccles J (1977) *The Self and its Brain.* Routledge and Kegan Paul, London.

Price J (1967) Hypothesis: the dominance hierarchy and the evolution of mental illness. *Lancet.* **2**: 243–66.

Price J and Sloman L (1987) Depression as yielding behaviour: an animal model based upon Schjelderup-Ebbe's pecking order. *Ethology and Sociobiology.* 85–98.

Prinzhorn H (1995) *The Artistry of the Mentally Ill.* Springer-Verlag, New York.

Progoff I (1953) *Jung's Psychology and its Social Meaning.* Routledge and Kegan Paul, London.

Pye D (1968) *The Nature and Art of Workmanship*. Cambridge University Press, Cambridge.

Ramachandran V and Blakeslee S (1998) *Phantoms in the Brain. Human nature and the architecture of the mind*. Fourth Estate, London.

Read H (1960) *The Form of Things Unknown*. Faber and Faber, London.

Ridley M (1996) *The Origins of Virtue*. Viking, London.

Rose H and Rose S (2000) *Alas Poor Darwin. Arguments against evolutionary psychology*. Jonathan Cape, London.

Rose S (1993) *The Making of Memory*. Bantam, London

Rose S (2004) Essay, consciousness. In: R Gregory (ed.) *Oxford Companion to the Mind* (2e). Oxford University Press, Oxford

Rosenfield I (1993) *The Strange, Familiar and Forgotten*. Vintage, London.

Ryle G (1949) *The Concept of Mind*. Hutchinson, London.

Saunders P and Skar P (2001) Archetypes, complexes and self-organisation. *Journal of Analytical Psychology*. **46**(2): 255–313.

Schachter S and Singer J (1962) Cognitive, social and physiological determinants of emotional state. *Psychological Reviews*. **69**: 379–99.

Scholem G (1961) *Major Trends in Jewish Mysticism*. Schocken Books, New York.

Schrödinger E (1944) *What is Life?* Cambridge University Press, Cambridge.

Schrödinger E (1957) *Science and Humanism*. Cambridge University Press, Cambridge.

Searle J (1997) *The Mystery of Consciousness*. Granta Books, London.

Segerstrale U (2001) *Defenders of the Truth: the sociobiology debate*. Oxford University Press, Oxford.

Shah S (1968) *The Way of the Sufi*. Jonathan Cape, London.

Shapiro G (1995) *Earthwards*. University of California Press, Berkley.

Sherrington C (1906) *Integrative Action of the Nervous System*. Yale University Press, New Haven (1961).

Simeon D and Abugel J (2006) *Feeling Unreal*. Oxford University Press, Oxford.

Sims A, Mundt C, Berner P and Barocka A (2000) In: M Gelder, J Lopez-Ibor and N Andreasen (eds) *New Oxford Textbook of Psychiatry*. Chapter 1.9. Oxford University Press, Oxford.

Slavin O and Kriegman D (1992) *The Adaptive Design of the Human Psyche*. Guilford Press, New York.

Smithson R (1979) Entropy and the new monuments. In: N Hort (ed.) *The Writings of Robert Smithson*. New York University Press, New York.

Southerington F (1971) *Hardy's Vision of Man*. Chatto and Windus, London.

Stafford-Clark D (1983) *What Freud Really Said*. Penguin, London.

Steele E, Lindley R and Blanden R (1998) *Lamarck's Signature*. Allen and Unwin, Sydney.

Steinberg D (1983) *The Clinical Psychiatry of Adolescence: clinical work from a social and developmental perspective*. Wiley, Chichester.

Steinberg D (1989) *Interprofessional Consultation*. Blackwell, Oxford.

Steinberg D (1992) Informed consent: consultation as a basis for collaboration between disciplines and between professionals and their patients. *Journal of Interprofessional Care*. 61: 43–8.

Steinberg D (2000) *Letters from the Clinic*. Routledge, London.

Steinberg D (2004a) From archetype to impressions: the magic of words. In: G Bolton, S Howlett, C Lago and J Wright (eds) *Writing Cures*. Brunner Routledge, London.

Steinberg D (2004b) Child and adolescent psychiatry: a model for medical teaching? *Journal of the Royal Society of Medicine*. 97: 545–6.

Steinberg D (2005) *Complexity in Healthcare and the Language of Consultation: exploring the other side of medicine*. Radcliffe Publishing, Oxford.

Stevens A (1982) *Archetype. A natural history of the self*. Routledge and Kegan Paul, London.

Stevens A (1990) *On Jung*. Routledge, London.

Stevens A (1993) *The Two Million Year Old Self*. A&M University Press, Texas.

Stevens A (2002) *Archetype Revisited. An updated natural history of the self*. Brunner Routledge, London.

Stevens A and Price J (1996) *Evolutionary Psychiatry*. Routledge, London.

Stilgoe J (1964) Foreword. In: G Bachelard (1964) *The Poetics of Space*. Orion, New York.

Storr A (1989) *Freud*. Oxford University Press, Oxford.

Storr A (ed.) (1998) *The Essential Jung*. Fontana, London.

Sulloway F (1979) *Freud: Biologist of the Mind – Beyond the Psychoanalytic Legend*. Burnett Books/André Deutsch, London.

Sumner R (1981) *Thomas Hardy, Psychological Novelist*. Macmillan, London

Sussman R (2006) Annual Conference of the American Association for the Advancement of Science, Washington University, St Louis, Missouri.

Sutherland S (1995) Consciousness. In: S Sutherland (ed.) *The International Dictionary of Psychology* (2e). Macmillan, London.

Tarkovsky A (1986) *Sculpting in Time. Reflections on the cinema*. The Bodley Head, London.

Tarkovsky A (1987) The apocalypse. *Temenos*. 8: 9–24.

Taylor D (1972) Psychiatry and sociology in the understanding of epilepsy. In: B Mandelbrot and G Gelder (eds) *Psychiatric Aspects of Medical Practice*. Staples, London

Thevoz M (1976) *Art Brut*. Skira, Geneva.

Thorne N (2000) *In Search of Martha Brown*. Dashwood Press, Sturminster Newton, Dorset.

Tinbergen N (1951) *The Study of Instinct*. Oxford University Press, London.

Tinbergen N (1953) *Social Behaviour in Animals*. Methuen, London.

Turovskaya M (1989) *Tarkovsky: cinema as poetry*. Faber and Faber, London.

Tyrer P (2002) Nidotherapy: a new approach to the treatment of personality disorder. *Acta Psychiatrica Scandinavica*. 105: 469–71.

Tyrer P and Bajaj P (2005) Nidotherapy: making the environment do the therapeutic work. *Advances in Psychiatric Treatment*. 11: 232–238.

Tyrer P and Steinberg D (2005) *Models for Mental Disorder: conceptual models in psychiatry* (4e). John Wiley, London.

Underhill E (1961) *Mysticism*. EP Dutton, New York.

Von Bertalanffy L (1968) *General Systems Theory*. George Braziller, New York.

Whitehead AN (1947) *Adventures of Ideas*. Cambridge University Press, Cambridge.

Williams J (1992) Eyes outside and eyes inside. In: M Tuchman and C Eliel (eds) *Parallel Visions*. Princeton University Press and Los Angeles County Museum of Art, Los Angeles. pp.14–15.

Wilson E (1979) *On Human Nature*. Bantam, New York.

Wilson E (1992) *The Diversity of Life*. Penguin, London.

Wilson FA (1958) *Art into Life*. Centaur Press, Sussex.

Wilson FA (1963) *Art as Understanding*. Routledge and Kegan Paul, London.

Wilson FA (1981) *Art as Revelation*. Centaur Press, Sussex.

Winnicott D (1972) *The Maturational Process and the Facilitating Environment*. Hogarth Press, London.

Wollheim R (1971) *Freud*. Fontana, London

Wolpert L (2006) *Six Impossible Things Before Breakfast*. Faber, London

Wood D (1992) *Derrida: a critical reader*. Blackwell, Oxford.

Wyss D (1966) *Depth Psychology: a critical history*. George Allen and Unwin, London.

Index

2001 (Kubrick) 33, 57

adrenalin 72, 104
adult attachment dynamic 81–2
aesthetics 26, 52, 132, 133, 143, 148
Aitchison, J 130
alphabet grid 30, 178
alternative medicine 171
altruism 130
ambiguity 12, 50–1, 121, 127, 181
amoeba 12, 70–2, 82, 142, 149, 153, 159
ancient wisdom 110, 180
Andre Rublev (Tarkovsky) 136
Andrea del Sarto (Browning) 47
animal awareness (primary consciousness) 152, 158, 159, 164, 175
animal behaviour
    archetypes 103
    arts 118, 130–1, 132
    attachment theory 63–4, 67–8, 69–72, 73, 74, 177
    consciousness of 3–4, 149, 152
    constituents of consciousness 55–6, 58–9, 141–3
    contribution to knowledge 10, 13
    group behaviour 48, 49
    mechanism for Io 154, 157
    sense of self 22, 145
    unconscious mind 141, 143
animal self (AS) 159, 160, 161, 162
anorexia nervosa 169
anthropic principle 96–7, 102, 106, 124, 129, 177, 185
anticipation
    art 119
    attachment theory 11, 80, 85, 88

autobiographical self 153
    evolution 142
    unconscious mind 176
anxiety 34–5, 61, 64, 83
apes 113, 130, 131 *see also* primates
archetypes 102–16
    arts 26, 119, 124, 131–2, 134, 138
    attachment theory 83–5, 88
    birth of 113–16
    collective unconscious 107–9
    constituents of consciousness 58, 103–7, 140
    cultural evolution 95
    definition 102–3
    evolution and self 111–13
    imagery 13–14, 20
    intuition and imagination 109–10
    mechanism for Io 154–5, 158, 160, 164, 165
    physicists' perspective 96
    Plato's cave 98
    self and brain 146
    unconscious mind 144, 145
    universe and mind 175, 182, 184
Aristotle 124
Arnheim, R 144, 145
arousal 72–4, 142
art(s) and artists 117–38
    aesthetics 148
    archetypes 112
    artist as explorer and leader 128–9
    attachment theory 63, 67, 69, 85, 87
    constituents of consciousness 140, 141
    and culture 119–23
    and curiosity 126–8

defining consciousness vi, 15–18, 118–19
definitions 1, 20, 25–6, 27, 117–18
   health education 173
   illusions 8, 9
   language 33, 130–1
   networks 125–6
   overview 137–8
   place 131–6, 161
   primitive imagery 11, 13
   and science 27, 41, 96, 123–5
   sense of self 23, 26
   society and politics 136–7
   unconscious mind 143, 144
   universe, religion and mind 123–5, 178, 180, 182, 183
artefacts
   arts 20, 26, 118, 135
   attachment theory 70, 87
   constituents of consciousness 140
   neuroscience 15
AS *see* animal self
asexual reproduction 62
atheism 90, 93
attachment theory 60–89
   adult attachment dynamic 81–2
   archetypes 83–5, 103–5, 112–13
   arousal 72–4
   connections 62–3
   cultural evolution 93, 95
   culture into mind 87–9
   defining consciousness 10, 55, 56
   definition 64–6
   dispositions to culture 86–7
   example 74–80
   Freud and followers 66–9
   language 131
   mechanism for Io 159
   overview 18, 19–20, 175, 177
   strange situations 60–1
   unconscious mind 70–2, 141
attractiveness 40, 41

autism spectrum disorder 86–7, 121, 129
autobiographical self 153, 154
awareness
   animals 152, 158, 159, 164, 175
   archetypes 111
   attachment theory 69, 83
   constituents of consciousness 55, 56, 168
   imagery 30, 31
   Kleinian theory 12
   mechanism for Io 157, 158, 161, 162, 163
   mind 142, 143, 148
   sense of self 22, 23, 25, 146
Ayer, AJ 176

Babel 45, 47–9, 50, 63, 135
babies *see* infants
Bachelard, G 135
Bahn, P 126
The Balcony (Genet) 99, 110
Barfield, Owen 175
Baron-Cohen, Simon 86
Barrow, J 96, 124
Barthes, R 99
basal ganglia 71
Bateson, Gregory 17, 18
Baudrillard, Jean 99
beauty 40, 136
Before Adam (London) 83
behavioural psychology 17, 34, 67, 111
being 154, 182
belief 18, 127, 141, 179, 181, 182, 184
Benn, Tony 110
Bennett, Alan 99
Berger, P 99
Berkeley, George 29, 95, 97, 182
Bible 27
'big art' 26, 117
Big Bang 22, 183
binding problem 146, 149, 152

biology vi, 9, 10, 13, 16, 17
bipolar disorder 129
birds 71–2, 118, 130, 142–3, 152, 159
Birdwhistell, R 133
Blackmore, S 26, 70
Blake, William 122
Blakeslee, Sandra 106, 139, 146–7
'blank slate' theory 87, 105
Block, N 24
Bloom, Harold 69
body 90–4, 147–50, 168, 179
Bohm, D 100, 143
Bohr, Neils 46, 58, 100, 118
Bolton, D 39
Booker, C 13
Boorstin, D 70
Bowlby, John 10, 60, 61, 64, 73, 79
brain
    archetypes 58, 107, 109, 111, 112
    arts 20, 26, 120, 127, 129, 130, 133
    attachment theory 69, 71, 73–4, 83, 87–9, 141
    constituents of consciousness 19, 56, 58
    cultural evolution 94, 95
    and culture 35–7
    group behaviour 45, 52
    illusions 8, 9
    inner and outer reality 29, 30
    language 33, 42, 176
    mechanism for Io 150, 151, 160–4, 175
    mind 28, 35–7, 40–1, 95, 142, 148–9
    neuroscience 10, 15, 24, 25
    physicists' perspective 96
    precognition 178–9
    sense of self 24–8, 139, 145–7
    size 56, 130, 133, 141
    unconscious mind 141, 143, 144, 145
Brain journal 66

Breton, André 121
Brooke, R 11
Brown, JAC 11, 12, 68
Browning, Robert 47
Buddha 27
Burnshaw, S 13

Campbell, Joseph 128
caretakers
    archetypes 104
    attachment 64, 74, 76, 78, 82, 88
    mechanism for Io 160, 161
caretaking behaviour (CB) 76
carousel image 4–5, 56, 95, 164–5
Carter, R 7, 24
Cartesian Theatre 150, 156
cartoons 99
categorising brain 9, 15, 19, 49, 112, 152
cathedrals 126, 137, 161
cautionary tales 19, 49
cave-paintings 126
CB (caretaking behaviour) 76
Chalmers, David 139, 148
children *see also* infants
    archetypes 109, 113
    attachment theory 64, 75, 76, 78
    healthcare 172
    mechanism for Io 155, 159
    psychiatry 170
    trauma 64
Chomsky, Noam 106
Christian Mysticism 27
cinema *see also* films
    archetypes 109
    civilisations 137
    definition of arts 25
    mechanism for Io 151, 156, 161, 163, 165
    neuroscience 15
    place and time 135
circularity *see* cyclical models
civilisation 120, 136, 137, 181
Clocksin, W 45

cloning 62
clowns 120, 128
collective unconscious 20, 107–9,
    119, 176
Collins, Cecil 122
communication 125, 126, 127
complementary medicine 171
complexity 34, 52, 85, 129, 151
computers
    mechanism for Io 146, 148, 150,
        151
    metaphor for mind 7, 10, 14, 26,
        49
    prediction 179
    unconscious mind 143
confidence 6, 38, 75, 77, 80, 81
conscience 83, 141
consciousness
    archetypes 85, 103–5, 116, 140
    arts 117–20, 131–3, 138, 140
    attachment theory 67, 69, 85, 89,
        141
    clinical practice 168–74
    connecting up 139–67
        constituents of
            consciousness 140–3,
            154–5
        Dennett, Edelman and
            Damasio 150–4
        dualism 147–50
        mechanism for Io 156–65
        self and brain 145–7
        self-awareness 139–40
        unconscious mind 143–5
    consciousness *by* 14, 32, 85
    consciousness disconnected
        22–44
        complexity 34–5
        culture 35–7
        evolution 40–1
        imagery and observer 31–2
        inner and outer reality 28–31
        language 33, 42
        mythology 33–4

philosophy 39
sense of self 22–8
systems models 37–8
tools for the trip 42–4
consciousness *of* 15, 32, 85
defining the subject 1–21
    archetypal imagery 13–14
    carousel metaphor 4–7
    differing approaches 7–11,
        14–18
    I, consciousness, self and
        soul 3–4
    overview vi, 1–3, 18–21
    primitive imagery 11–13
how chemicals become
    conscious 53–9
physicists' perspective 96–7
Schrödinger's cat 97–8
tribal behaviour 50, 52
in whose image? 175–85
    creativity 180–1
    Erikson 181–2
    language 175–7
    precognition 178–9
    religion and spirituality
        176–8, 181, 183–5
    universe and mind 182–5
consultative work 171–3
conviction 33, 34, 127, 136, 184,
    185
Cooramaswamy, AK 117
core self 153, 154
cortex 71, 146, 151, 164
Creation 165–6
The Creation (Haydn) 46
Creation Out of Nothing (Cupitt) 176
creationism 7, 93
creativity
    arts 25, 27, 118, 128, 129
    attachment theory 63, 70, 74
    as challenge 48
    constituents of consciousness 57,
        140, 155, 164
    defining consciousness 15, 16, 18

illusions 8
intuition 180
prediction 179
primitive imagery 13
Crick, Francis 139, 146, 147
Critchley, McDonald 29
Crompton, Richmal 44
cultural self (CS) 160, 161, 162
culture
    archetypes 140
    arts 20, 26, 27, 119–23, 126, 136
    attachment theory 69, 70, 85,
        86–9, 141
    constituents of
        consciousness 35–7, 57–8,
        140–2
    cultural evolution 28, 93, 94–5
    language 33, 42
    mechanism for Io 160, 165
    memory 93, 164
    sense of self 25–8, 30
    tribal behaviour 47, 48–9, 52
    unconscious mind 141, 143, 144
    universe and mind 175, 176, 180,
        182
Cupitt, Don 176–7, 181, 184
curiosity 13, 111, 124, 126–8, 132,
    155
cyclical models
    archetypes 20
    arts 118, 124
    attachment theory 64, 65, 66
    carousel metaphor 4, 5, 56
    relationships 37–8
    sense of self 152, 158
    universe and mind 185

Damasio, Antonio 23, 32, 139,
    152–4, 156, 158, 161
Darwinian theory 53, 93, 151, 152,
    185
Davies, P 96
Dawkins, Richard 26, 39, 40, 70, 75,
    93, 182

death 125, 134, 181
deception 50–1, 56, 57, 69, 130, 141
defence mechanisms 67
de Kooning, Willem 122
delusions 168, 185
denial 67, 69
Dennett, Daniel
    consciousness 8, 58
    dualism 91
    mechanism for Io 32, 156, 161
    mind 150–1
    self-awareness 139
    sense of self 23, 24
depersonalisation 163, 168
depression 12, 64, 73, 112, 131
'depth' psychology 25, 66
Derrida, Jacques 99
Descartes, René 90, 147
development
    archetypes 111, 113
    arts 131
    attachment theory 10, 69, 72,
        75–6, 78, 87–8
    brain/mind 27–8, 30, 69, 71–2,
        87, 151
    culture 28, 35–7, 69, 88, 93–5
    defining consciousness 2
    Kleinian theory 12, 13
    Lacan 158
dialectical materialists 122
Dickinson, Emily 123
disorders 5, 86–7, 112, 128–9, 155,
    168–70, 173
dispositions 86–7, 153
diversity 62, 129, 151
DNA (deoxyribonucleic acid) 92, 93,
    105, 185
Donne, John 90, 95
drama 25, 46, 88, 99, 137
dreams
    archetypes 108
    arts 128, 135
    attachment theory 67, 141
    illusions 9–10

imagery 11, 12, 32
intuition 34
drugs 170, 180
dualism 9, 90, 91, 92, 147–50
Dubuffet, Jean 1, 17

Eccles, John 139, 145
Eckhart, Meister 27
Edelman, G 15, 32, 94, 139, 151–2,
    154, 161
Eden 19, 45, 46–7
editing model (Dennett) 150, 151
education 98, 173–4
ego 68, 84, 181, 182
Ehrenzweig, A 143
Eight and a Half (Fellini) 162–3
emerging mind/brain 12, 13, 27,
    111, 112, 136
emotion *see* feelings
empathy 57–8, 83, 85, 86, 121, 130,
    141
energy 4–7, 183
'Entropy and the new monuments'
    (Smithson) 134
Erikson, Erik 181, 182
ESP (extra-sensory perception) 179
ethology 20, 35, 64, 111, 131
evolution
    archetypes 84–5, 88, 103, 108,
        111–13, 140
    arts 26–7, 127, 128, 130–1, 132,
        133
    attachment theory 60–2, 64,
        71–2, 74, 80, 84–5, 88
    constituents of
        consciousness 33–4, 39–42,
        44, 140–2
    culture 28, 35–7, 93, 94–5
    defining consciousness vi, 2, 6–7,
        12, 19, 20
    Edelman 151, 152
    how chemicals become
        conscious 53–9
    mechanism for Io 158, 159

memory 92, 93, 94
    sense of self 26, 27, 28
    tribal behaviour 47, 52
    universe and mind 175, 184, 185
evolutionary biology 10, 17
evolutionary psychology 16, 17
experiential selection 151
exploration 74–7, 78–9, 80, 81, 111,
    132
extra-sensory perception (ESP) 179
Ey, Henri 66

faces
    archetypes 109, 110, 113
    beauty 40
    binding problem 146
    first human face 177
    hollow mask experiment 73
    mechanism for Io 158, 159
fairground image 4–7, 95, 161, 162
faith 136, 178
family 64–6, 130
fantasy
    archetypes 85, 88, 113
    arts 121–4, 126–9
    attachment theory 10, 19, 66–7,
        80–1, 85, 88, 141
    imagery 11, 176, 180
    imagination 140
    intuition 34
    tribal behaviour 52
fear 35, 56, 81, 127, 129, 136
feelings
    archetypes 113
    arts 124, 129, 132
    attachment theory 10–11, 62, 81,
        83, 86, 141
    constituents of consciousness 37,
        55–7, 142, 176
    mechanism for Io 158
    sense of self 24
    unconscious mind 144
Fellini, Federico 9, 129, 162, 163,
    181

fight, fright, flight 74, 103, 113, 136
films *see also* cinema
    archetypes 88
    arts 25–6, 117, 122, 135, 136, 137
    folklore 19
    illusions 9–10
    language 33
    mechanism for Io 156, 162–3
    neuroscience 15
    projection 57
Fitzpatrick, M 174
folklore
    archetypes 108
    arts 123, 137
    cautionary tales 18, 19
    precognition 179
    primitive imagery 11, 13
    tribal behaviour 45, 47
fools 120, 122, 136, 137
Forster, EM 62
Foucault, M 67
Fowles, John 133
fractals 111, 185
free association 121
free will 149
Freud, Sigmund
    academic dissent 16
    arts 26, 122, 136
    attachment theory 10, 66–9, 79
    clinical practice 170
    constituents of consciousness 54,
        58, 141–3, 149, 157
    postmodernism 100
    psychodynamic theory 11
    psychology 25
Furedi, F 174

Gabo, Naum 121
Garden of Eden 19, 45, 46–7
Gazzaniga, Michael 139, 146
genes
    archetypes 14, 111, 112, 115, 116
    attachment theory 62, 87, 141
    Damasio 153

defining consciousness 3, 10,
    16–18, 20
    Edelman 151
    how chemicals become
        conscious 53–9, 142
    memory and body 92, 93
    Schrödinger's cat 97
    tribal behaviour 52
Genet, Jean 85, 99, 110
geological model 107, 143
Gerhart, J 53
gestalt theory 51, 143, 144, 145
Gladwell, M 129
The Glassblowers (Peake) 182
Glyn-Jones, Anne 137
Gnosticism 184
God/gods
    archetypes 14
    arts 118, 123, 136
    mythology 33
    primitive imagery 12
    universe, religion and mind 90,
        166, 176, 178, 183–5
Godel's theorem 148
Goethe, Johann Wolfgang von 27,
    128
Golding, William 83
Goldman, A 24
'good enough' 11, 82, 142
Gould, Stephen Jay 92, 93
Graham, Gordon 179, 180
'grappling hook' analogy 57, 87–8,
    118, 122, 125, 134, 178
gravitational OR (objective
    reduction) 149
gravity 77, 149, 183, 185
Greenfield, S 24
Gregory, Richard 28, 73
grief 73, 131
group behaviour 48–9, 50, 84, 85,
    130
gut feelings 110, 164
Güzeldere, G 7, 24

hallucinations 32, 126, 146
Hardy, Thomas 27, 133–4
Haydn, Joseph 46
healthcare 168, 170, 171, 172, 173–4
Heerwagen, J 132
Hegel, GWF 135
Heidegger, Martin 46
Heil, J 39
Hepburn, J 132–3
heroes 85, 110
higher order consciousness 152
Hinduism 27
Hinshelwood, RD 11
hippocampus 164
Hitler, Adolf 110
Hofstadter, Douglas 14, 139, 146
'Holding up a Mirror' (Glyn-Jones) 137
'hollow mask' experiment (Gregory) 73
holy fool 136, 137
Horrobin, David 123, 129
Howard's End (Forster) 62
humanism 176
humanities 25, 27
humans
    archetypes 20, 107
    arts 118, 129, 130
    attachment theory 10, 60
    faces 177
    how chemicals become conscious 56–9
    human nature 11, 145
    sense of self 3, 23
humour 99, 120, 121, 181
Humphrey, Nicholas 15, 139, 149
Huxley, Aldous 180

'I'
    archetypes 84, 106
    arts 124, 136
    attachment theory 68, 84

defining consciousness vi, 3–5, 8, 20, 59
    dualism 147, 149
    mechanism for Io 159–61, 162–5
    self and brain 145, 146, 147, 150
    self-awareness 139
    unconscious mind 144
    universe and mind 175, 181, 183
Id 12, 67, 68
idealists 91, 92, 147
ideas
    archetypes 108
    arts 118
    attachment theory 70
    defining consciousness 5, 15
    natural and supernatural 180
    projection 57
    tribal behaviour 48
identification with other 158, 159
identity
    attachment theory 65, 84
    babies 157
    carousel metaphor 6
    mechanism for Io 161, 162
    memory 153
    sense of self 20, 22
ideologies 33, 48, 140
illusions
    ambiguity 51
    arts 126, 136
    attachment theory 70, 73
    defining consciousness 8–10, 17, 18, 176
    self and brain 147
imagery
    archetypes 13–14, 88–9, 108–10, 111–15
    arts 25, 119–21, 124–6, 140
    attachment theory 60–1, 70, 72, 76, 79–80, 84, 88–9
    constituents of consciousness 28, 30–2, 34–5, 140–1, 152, 154
    defining consciousness 1–2, 10, 16, 19, 20

how chemicals become
   conscious 55, 56, 57, 59
mechanism for Io 156, 157, 162
postmodernism 100
primitive imagery 11–13
tribal behaviour 52
universe and mind 176, 185
imagination
   archetypes 85, 88, 109–10, 112,
      113
   arts 26, 127, 135
   attachment theory 66, 70, 74, 85,
      88
   defining consciousness 10, 18
   how chemicals become
      conscious 57
   mechanism for Io 162
   and reality 140–1
   religion 178
   tribal behaviour 45
immune response 93, 151
infants
   archetypes 104–5, 109, 110, 112,
      113
   attachment theory 64, 72–8, 82,
      88, 141
   cultural evolution 95
   dualism 149
   human face 177
   mechanism for Io 157, 158, 159
   universe and mind 182
information technology 14, 143
The Inheritors (Golding) 83
inhibitions 83
inner imagery
   archetypes 103, 111, 113
   arts 126
   attachment theory 10, 60, 76, 79,
      80, 84
   how chemicals become
      conscious 56
   primitive imagery 11
   tribal behaviour 52
inner reality 28–31

innovation 57, 63, 93, 128
insight 25, 100, 148
instincts
   archetypes 83, 103, 108, 111
   arts 120, 124
   constituents of
      consciousness 142, 158
   primitive imagery 11
intelligent design 183, 184, 185
internal working image 79–80
Internet 179–80
introjected good parent 80, 82
introspection 66
intuition
   archetypes 109–10
   arts 135, 136
   attachment theory 66
   defining consciousness 34
   dualism 148
   universe and mind 165, 179, 180,
      181, 184
Io (observing 'I')
   arts 125
   attachment theory 76, 84
   cinema metaphor 156–7, 165
   components of 159–61
   constituents of
      consciousness 150, 153, 154
   how chemicals become
      conscious 59
   imagery 31–2, 163
   Lacan 157–9
   memory 162, 163–4
   physicists' perspective 96
   self and brain 146
   universe and mind 176, 180
Islam 27, 178

Jacobi, J 107
James, Henry 27
James, William 27, 143
James-Lange hypothesis 120
Jaspers, Karl 27, 168, 169, 170
Jaynes, Julian 32, 139, 146

jesters 120
Jewish mysticism 165, 183
Johnson, Mark 78–9
jokes 99
Jung, CG
    archetypes 13–14, 58, 102,
       107–9, 111–12, 116
    arts 120, 122, 124, 134
    attachment theory 68
    defining consciousness 16, 20
    mechanism for Io 154, 157
    Plato's cave 98
    primitive imagery 11, 13
    psychology 25

Kabbalah 27, 183
Kandinsky, W 121, 124
Kinesics and Context
    (Birdwhistell) 133
Kipling, Rudyard 46, 180, 184
Kirschner, M 53
Klein, Melanie 11, 12, 68
Kleinian theory 11–12, 16, 25, 41,
    48, 68
knowing 135, 154
knowledge 19, 46–7, 83, 128, 135,
    153
Knox, Jean 60, 103, 109, 111–13,
    116
Kriegman, D 82
Kübler, George 135
Kubrick, Stanley 33, 57

Lacan, Jacques 68, 79, 157–9
Lamarck, Jean-Baptiste de 20, 92
Lamarckism 93, 94, 108, 112, 164
landscape 131–3
Langer, Susanne 119, 120
language
    archetypes 58, 84–5, 103, 106,
       113, 116
    arts 118, 130–1, 133, 140
    attachment theory 69, 79, 84, 85,
       88

constituents of consciousness 33,
    39, 57–8, 140, 142, 155
    mechanism for Io 158, 164
    memory 94, 164
    postmodernism 100
    primitive imagery 13
    self and brain 145, 146
    tribal behaviour 46, 50
    unconscious mind 144, 145
    universe and mind 175–8, 183,
       184
laws of universe 3, 125, 165, 183,
    185
Leach, E 48
learning 62, 113, 132, 143, 146, 160,
    174
Leja, M 122
Lem, Stanislau 136
Leon, Moses de 27
Levin, D 94
Lévi-Strauss, C 106
Lewis-Williams, David 126
limbic system 71, 164
linearity 4, 9, 38, 39, 64, 66
Lipowski, Z 168
literature 9, 13, 27, 137, 145, 164,
    173
Lodge, David 27
London, Jack 83, 136
long-term memory 164
Lorenz, K 142
loss 64, 73, 131, 134
Luckman, T 99
Luria, A 144
Lyons, J 116

MacLean, P 71
The Madness of King George
    (Bennett) 99
Magritte, René 98
Malik, Kenan 145
Malraux, A 135
mammals 71, 72, 152, 159
Mandelbrot, B 55, 63

Maritain, Jaques 124
Marx, Karl 100
materialists 91, 92, 122, 147, 148,
    182
mathematics 14, 53, 111–12, 148–9,
    182–3
McCrone, J 133, 139
McDowell, M 112
ME (myalgic
    encephalomyelitis) 169
meanings
    archetypes 112
    arts 127
    attachment theory 60, 72
    constituents of consciousness 35,
        42–4
    health education 173
    Lacan 158
    language 33, 42, 176
    postmodernism 98
    religion 177
    tribal behaviour 52
    unconscious mind 143, 144
medical model 170, 171
medicine 4, 169, 170, 171
meiosis (sexual reproduction) 62, 63
memes 26, 70, 87, 94, 118, 165
memory
    archetypes 84–5, 88, 109, 113,
        140
    arts 131, 133, 135, 136
    attachment theory 10–11, 60, 70,
        72, 80, 84–5, 88
    and body 92–4
    constituents of
        consciousness 140–2, 150,
        152, 153
    defining consciousness 9, 13, 16
    how chemicals become
        conscious 55, 56
    mechanism for Io 32, 157, 160,
        162, 163, 164
    self-awareness 139
    tribal behaviour 45, 52

unconscious mind 70, 72, 145
universe and mind 175, 176, 178,
    180
mental health 21, 48, 168, 169–71
metaphors
    archetypes 112
    arts 25, 26, 135
    attachment theory 69, 72, 88
    language 33, 42, 155
    mechanism for Io 158, 164
    memory 94
    postmodernism 100
    unconscious mind 58, 143, 145
    universe and mind 182
Meyer, S 185
Milton, John 46
mimicry 158
mind
    archetypes 102, 103, 108, 116
    arts 20, 26–7, 118–19, 124, 130,
        136, 138
    attachment theory 19, 60–1,
        67–72, 87–9
    constituents of
        consciousness 35–7, 39, 41,
        140, 142, 150, 154
    defining consciousness 8, 12–13,
        15–17, 20–1
    definition 28
    dualism 90–2, 147–50
    how chemicals become
        conscious 57, 59
    language 42
    mechanism for Io 156, 158, 160
    memory 94
    neuroscience 15, 25
    self and brain 145, 146, 147
    self-awareness 139
    tribal behaviour 46, 52
    unconscious 70–2, 143–5
    universe and religion 95–6, 177,
        178, 180, 182–5
Mirror (Tarkovsky) 136
mirrors 158, 161, 162, 163

Mnemosyne 4, 32, 164
Mondrian, Piet 121
monism 90, 91, 92, 147
monsters 88, 108, 115, 116
monuments 134, 135
Moore, Henry 120, 121
mother figure
    archetypes 14, 105, 108–10, 112,
        113
    attachment theory 64, 72, 73,
        74–5, 79, 88
    human face 177
    imagery 12, 14
    memory 160
'movie in the brain' (Damasio) 152,
    156
multiple drafts model (Dennett) 150
Murphy, Todd 178
music 25, 117, 119, 120, 123, 137,
    182
myalgic encephalomyelitis
    (ME) 169
mysticism 14, 27, 165, 183, 184
mythology
    archetypes 115
    arts 25, 128, 129, 135, 138
    attachment theory 69, 141
    constituents of consciousness 27,
        33–4, 37, 58, 151
    imagination and reality 140
    language 33
    mechanism for Io 161, 165
    primitive imagery 11, 13
    tribal behaviour 45, 47

narcissism 177, 181
narratives
    archetypes 84, 108, 116, 140
    arts 25–7, 129, 137, 138, 140
    defining consciousness 13, 18,
        150, 155
    language 33, 42
    memory 164
    religion 178

sense of self 25
tribal behaviour 45, 46, 47,
    52
natural selection 70
nature 90, 136, 175
Nazi regimes 137
neglect 6, 64, 77, 177
nerve cells *see* neurones
nervous system
    archetypes 88, 105, 110, 116
    dualism 149
    how chemicals become
        conscious 6, 55, 57
    mechanism for Io 152, 153,
        161
    universe and mind 182, 185
Neural Darwinism 151
neural network
    arts 126, 138
    constituents of
        consciousness 139, 146, 151,
        152, 154
    dualism 149
    mechanism for Io 160, 164
    universe and mind 175, 178
neurobiology 26, 148
neurones
    attachment theory 67
    constituents of consciousness
        5, 14, 30, 41, 146, 151
    dualism 148, 149
    unconscious mind 143, 144
neuroscience
    archetypes 14, 58, 103, 109
    defining consciousness 9, 10,
        14–16, 146, 150, 164
    sense of self 24
neurosis 26, 68, 141
Nostalgia (Tarkovsky) 136
not-self 159
novelists 13, 17, 41, 133
Nunn, C 169
nurturing behaviour 55, 56, 71, 72,
    77, 160

object relations 103, 153
objectivity
 ambiguity 51
 arts 20, 41, 121
 attachment theory 66
 defining consciousness 18
 intuition 34
 physicists' perspective 96
On the Spiritual in Art
  (Kandinsky) 124
Organic Memory (Otis) 164
Orians, G 132
Orosius 137
'other' 123, 158, 159, 162
Otis, Laura 94, 145, 164
outer reality 28–31
'outsider' artists 122
Oxford Textbook of Psychiatry 168

Pagels, H 97
Paglia, Camille 123, 136
panpsychism 148
pantheism 90
Paradise Lost (Milton) 46
'Paradoxes and Problems'
  (Donne) 90
paranoia 12–13, 58, 74, 115, 128,
  141, 179
Parkes, Colin 73, 131
past 109, 133, 153
PC (political correctness) 173–4
Peake, Mervyn 182
Penrose, Roger 139, 148, 149, 151,
  183, 185
perception
 arts 25, 132, 140
 attachment theory 10–11, 60, 73,
  74
 constituents of consciousness 29,
  40, 146, 150, 152
 defining consciousness 1–2, 13,
  16, 20
 dualism 148, 149
 memory 94

prediction 179
 sense of self 22, 25, 162
 tribal behaviour 52
personality 2, 27, 42, 64, 82, 87, 155
philosophy
 arts 133
 defining consciousness 14, 15,
  17, 27, 39
 health education 173
 mind and body 91, 95
 universe and mind 180, 182, 184
physics *see also* quantum physics
 arts 125
 clinical practice 168
 dualism 149
 physicists' perspective 95, 96–7
 Schrödinger's cat 97, 98
 unconscious mind 145
 universe 183
Picasso, Pablo 121
Pinker, Steven 94, 139, 144, 146,
  147
place, in arts 131–6
Plato
 archetypes 106, 111, 116
 arts 134
 attachment theory 69
 dualism 148
 Plato's cave 98
 science 27
The Poetics of Space (Bachelard) 135
poetry and poets 117–38
 archetypes 112
 art and consciousness 118–19
 art and curiosity 126–8
 art, expression, culture 119–23
 art, science, spirituality 41,
  123–5
 art, society, politics 136–7
 artist as explorer and leader
  128–9
 attachment theory 62
 defining arts 25–6, 117–18
 defining consciousness 16, 17

health education 173
illusions 8, 9
language 130–1
memory 164
networks 125–6
overview 137–8, 184
place 131–6
Plato's cave 98
primitive imagery 13
sense of self 23, 25–6, 27
tribal behaviour 45, 47
political correctness (PC) 173–4
politics 33, 69, 136–7
Pollock, Jackson 122
Popper, Karl 127, 139, 145
postmodernism 95, 98–9
'The prayer of Miriam Cohen'
(Kipling) 46
precognition 178–9
prediction 179
predispositions
attachment theory 64, 86, 88
defining consciousness 3, 5, 14,
176
physicists' perspective 96
tribal behaviour 52
prehension 40
Price, John 123, 128
primary consciousness 152
primates
archetypes 113
arts 130, 131, 137
attachment theory 68, 71, 72, 75
defining consciousness 4, 10, 159
schizophrenia 129
primitive imagery 11–13, 163
Princess of Wales 110
projection 57, 68, 69, 85, 89, 118
property dualists 91, 92, 147–8
proto-emotion 56, 74
proto-self 150, 152, 153, 154, 158,
175
protozoa 55, 62, 82, 103–4, 142, 143
Proust, Marcel 27, 149

proximity-seeking attachment
behaviour (PSAB) 76
psyche 25, 60, 110
psychiatry
archetypes 58, 103
attachment theory 64
clinical practice 168, 169, 170
defining consciousness xi, x, 4
physicists' perspective 96
psychoanalytic theory
arts 26, 121, 122, 127, 131
attachment theory 64, 66–9, 73,
80
clinical practice 170
defining consciousness 17, 153,
155, 180
intuition 34
postmodernism 98, 100
primitive imagery 11, 13
projection 57
psychology 25
psychodynamic theory
archetypes 13, 103
attachment theory 19, 61, 64, 66,
67, 68
defining consciousness vi, 10, 16,
58
primitive imagery 11–13
psychology 25
psychology
archetypes 103, 107–9
arts 27, 134
clinical practice 170, 171
defining consciousness 9, 10, 13,
16
definition 25
language 33
physicists' perspective 96
tribal behaviour 45, 49
unconscious mind 145
Pye, David 118

qualia 106, 115, 150
quantum indeterminism 149

quantum physics *see also* physics
  archetypes 106
  arts 125, 129
  defining consciousness 2, 153
  dualism 148
  mind makes world 95, 96
  postmodernism 100
  unconscious mind 143
  universe and mind 180, 183, 184

racialism 107
Ramachandran, VS 106, 139, 146–7
Read, H 120, 121
'real dreams' (Fellini) 9, 181
reality
  alternative realities 98–101
  ambiguity 51
  arts 121, 122, 123, 127, 136
  illusions 9
  imagination 140–1
  inner and outer reality 28–31, 44
  mythology 33
  philosophy 39
  physicists' perspective 96–7
  postmodernism 98–9, 100
  Schrödinger's cat 97
reciprocity 28, 30, 52, 64, 185
regression 44, 61, 69, 81, 155
relationships
  archetypes 103, 106
  arts 119, 136
  attachment theory 60, 63, 68, 70,
    74–5, 81–2, 85, 159
  constituents of consciousness 16,
    35, 37, 141, 145
  how chemicals become
    conscious 56, 58
  universe and mind 175, 176
religion
  arts 26, 126, 136
  defining consciousness 4, 18, 90,
    141
  sense of self 23, 26, 161
  tribal behaviour 45, 49, 51

universe and mind 176, 178, 181,
    183, 184
'remembered present'
  (Edelman) 152
Remembrance of Things Past
  (Proust) 149
repression 67
reproduction 52, 62, 81, 112
reptiles 49, 55, 71, 73, 105, 108, 152,
    159
Republic (Plato) 98
responsiveness 3, 23, 55, 157
Ridley, M 141
risk-taking 5, 6, 81–2
RNA (ribonucleic acid) 92, 185
roles 64, 65, 66, 84, 85
Rose, H 7, 17
Rose, S 7, 17, 164
Rosenfield, I 94
Rothko, Mark 122
Roti, Nino 163

Saddam Hussein 110
St Augustine 22, 30
Sandburg, Carl 45
sanity xi, 17–18, 33, 51–2, 100, 141
Saunders, P 111
savannah 132, 161
Schachter, S 72
schizophrenia 128, 129
Schrödinger, Erwin 97, 98
Schrödinger's cat 96, 97–8
science
  archetypes 111
  arts 123–5, 136
  attachment theory 63, 67, 87
  defining consciousness 4, 7, 8,
    14, 17, 18
  definition 27
  dualism 91
  health education 173, 174
  memory 164
  physicists' perspective 96
  sense of self 23, 27

tribal behaviour 46
unconscious mind 144
universe and mind 177, 180
Sculpting in Time (Tarkovsky) 135
Searle, John 7, 10, 14, 49, 91, 147–8,
   150
Segerstrale, U 7, 17
selection 70, 93, 96, 128, 151
self
   animal and cultural self 159–62
   archetypes 88, 111–13
   arts 27, 122, 123, 125, 133
   attachment theory 70, 88
   and brain 145–7
   defining consciousness 1, 3, 7,
      12, 19, 58, 155
   dualism 149, 150
   inner and outer reality 28, 30
   mechanism for Io 150, 152, 153,
      156–9, 161–3
   sense of 22–4, 27, 139
   universe and mind 175, 176, 180,
      181
self-awareness 3, 8–9, 23, 139–41,
   145–6
self-consciousness 3, 9, 20–4, 32, 89,
   154, 162
self-esteem 6, 66
self-identity 6, 20, 44, 65, 84
'selfish' gene 141
sentience 23, 58, 59, 146
Sexual Personae (Paglia) 136
sexual reproduction 62
sexuality 123, 136, 141
Shakespeare, William 27
The Shape of Time (Kübler) 135
Shapiro, Gary 135
Sherrington, C 11, 41, 113
short-term memory 164
signifiers 158
Sims, A 168
Singer, J 72
Skar, P 111
Smithson, Robert 134, 135

social biology 10, 16
The Social Construction of Reality
   (Berger and Luckman) 99
social psychology 15, 25
social science 7, 9, 16, 17, 18
social skills 43, 44, 52, 130
society, and arts 136–7
sociobiology 10, 16
Socrates 69, 106
Solaris (Tarkovsky) 136
songs 40, 130
soul vi, 4, 8, 90–1, 147, 184
Soviet regimes 137
space 160, 161
speech 119, 176
Spinoza, Benedict (Baruch) 27, 90,
   96
Spiral Jetty, Utah 134, 135
spirals 37, 124
spirit 91, 120, 124, 126, 143
spirituality
   arts 123–5, 127, 128, 136
   clinical practice 170
   science 27
   universe and mind 165, 176, 179,
      181
Stafford-Clark, D 11, 69
Stalker (Tarkovsky) 136
stereotypes 105, 119
Stevens, Anthony 107, 111, 123, 128
stories *see* narratives
Storr, A 11, 13, 68, 69, 107
strange situations 60–1, 78
stream of consciousness 150
stress 61, 81
subculture 35, 37, 70
subjectivity
   ambiguity 51
   archetypes 106
   arts 20, 41, 121
   attachment theory 66
   defining consciousness 9, 18, 37
   intuition 34
   psychology 25

sub-selves 163
substance dualists 91, 92, 147
Sufism 27
Sulloway, F 58, 69
Sumner, Rosemary 134
Super-ego 68
supernatural vi, 4, 179, 180
surrealism 98, 121, 122
survival
    archetypes 84–5, 88, 103–5, 111,
        112, 114
    arts 130
    attachment theory 60, 63–4,
        74–5, 77–8, 81–5, 88, 141
    constituents of consciousness 54,
        56, 57, 93, 151
    mechanism for Io 158, 159
    tribal behaviour 52
    universe and mind 177, 181
Sutherland, Stuart 7, 24
symbolism
    archetypes 84, 106, 111
    arts 25, 119, 140
    attachment theory 67, 70, 84, 88
    constituents of consciousness 58,
        155
    language 33, 106
    postmodernism 100
    unconscious mind 144, 145
    universe and mind 176, 178, 180,
        182–3
synapses 35–7, 129, 143, 151
systems models 37, 64

taboos 46, 62
tales see narratives
Tarkovsky, Andrey 135–6
tautologies 23, 24, 139
Taylor, David 182
teasing 121
thalamus 146, 151
theology 16, 17, 41, 176
theory of mind 86
Therapeutic Society 174

thought-experiments 53, 97, 98,
    106, 147
Three Dancers (Picasso) 121
time 41, 53, 62–3, 133–6, 160
Tinbergen, N 10, 142
Tipler, F 96
Tower of Babel 45, 47–9, 50, 63, 135
transference 68
Tree of Knowledge 19, 46, 83, 135
tribal behaviour 18, 45–50, 51, 52,
    130
triune brain 71
trust 58, 75, 141
truth 98
Tyrer, P 16, 64

uncertainty 10, 12, 97, 98, 127,
    184
unconscious
    archetypes 107–9, 111
    arts 120, 121, 124, 138
    attachment theory 19, 66, 67, 69,
        70–2, 74, 141
    constituents of consciousness 30,
        32, 35, 142, 143, 158
    defining consciousness 14, 20,
        101
    how chemicals become
        conscious 58, 59
    language 42
    locating 143–5
    mechanism for Io 155, 163
    neuroscience 15
    philosophy 39
    psychology 25, 100
    universe and mind 176, 178, 180
universe 96, 123–5, 145, 165,
    175–8, 180, 182–5

vertigo 29
Vigotsky, Lev 144
violence 83, 123, 137
virtual reality 9, 29, 30
visionaries 87, 122, 128, 134, 184

visual perception 29, 40, 146
vitalism 91

warnings 46, 47, 49, 81–2
wars 37, 181
The Well-Beloved (Hardy) 134
Wertheimer, Max 145
What is Life? (Schrödinger) 97
Whitehead, Alfred North 40
will 5, 6, 149
Wilson, Frank Avray 123
Winnicott, Donald 82, 127
Wollheim, R 69
Wolpert, Lewis 34
words
    archetypes 106
    arts 119, 130–1
    attachment theory 62, 70, 72

constituents of consciousness 42,
    155, 158
health education 173
narratives 46
projection 57
unconscious mind 143, 144,
    145
universe and mind 175, 176, 178,
    180, 182, 184
workmanship 118
writers
    art 26, 122, 125, 133, 135
    imagery 9, 11, 46, 176
    sense of self 23, 26, 27
Wyss, Dieter 25

Zohar 27, 165, 183, 184
'zombie' phenomenon 146

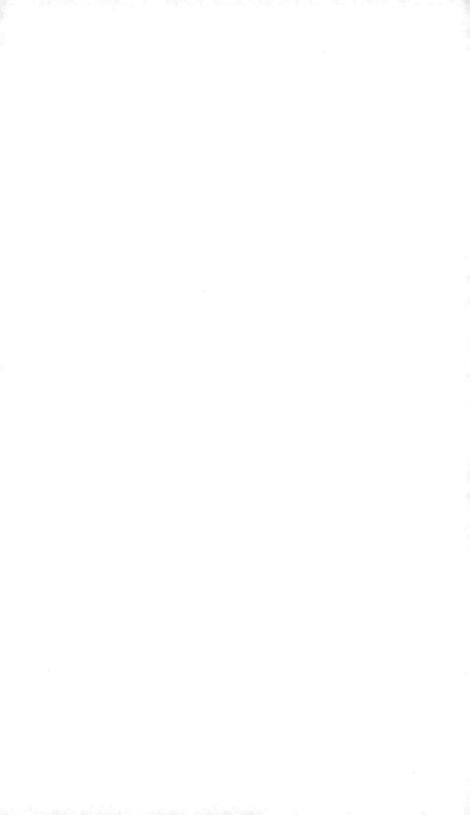